COMMUNITY CARE,

Learning Services

Please return
on or before
the last date
stamped below

CITY COLLEGE
NORWICH

1 6 MAR 2005	1 0 SEP 2010
- 8 NOV 2006	- 7 SEP 2011
2 9 NOV 2006	
0 8 JAN 2007	
1 7 APR 2007	
1 4 MAY 2007	
1 6 MAR 2009	
1 5 MAR 2010	
2 3 APR 2010	

CONTEMPORARY SOCIAL POLICY

Series Editor: Michael Sullivan, University of Wales, Swansea

A series of concise and accessible introductory guides to key topics and issues in contemporary social policy.

Also available in the series:

Ken Blakemore and Robert F. Drake
Understanding Equal Opportunity Policies

Ian Law
Racism, Ethnicity and Social Policy

COMMUNITY CARE, IDEOLOGY AND SOCIAL POLICY

HARRY COWEN
Cheltenham & Gloucester College of Higher Education

PRENTICE HALL EUROPE

London New York Toronto Sydney Tokyo
Singapore Madrid Mexico City Munich Paris

First published 1999 by
Prentice Hall Europe
Campus 400, Maylands Avenue
Hemel Hempstead
Hertfordshire, HP2 7EZ
A division of
Simon & Schuster International Group

Typeset in 10/12pt Baskerville by
Hands Fotoset, Ratby, Leicester

Printed and bound in Great Britain by
MPG Books Ltd, Bodmin, Cornwall

Library of Congress Cataloging-in-Publication Data

Cowen, Harry, 1942–
    Community care, ideology, and social policy / Harry Cowen.
        p.   cm. — (Contemporary social policy)
    Includes bibliographical references and index.
    ISBN 0–13–727843–8 (alk. paper)
    1. Home care services—Great Britain.   2. Aged—Home care—
Great Britain.   3. Handicapped—Home care—Great Britain.
4. Homeless persons—Care—Great Britain.   5. Mentally
handicapped—Care—Great Britain.   6. Caregivers—Great Britain.
7. Great Britain—Social policy.   I. Title   II. Series: Contemporary
social policy series.
    HV1481.G52C68   1998
    361.8'0941—dc21   98–5599
                                                                          CIP

British Library Cataloguing in Publication Data

A catalogue record for this book is available from
the British Library

ISBN 0–13–727843–8

1 2 3 4 5 6   02 01 00 99

To my daughter Carla,
and to the memory of
my father, Mark

CONTENTS

Series Editor's Preface   xi

Preface   xiii

Acknowledgements   xvi

**PART I SOCIAL POLICIES IN HEALTH AND
SOCIAL CARE**   **1**

1 Introduction: community, policy and ideology   **3**
Prime focus of the book   3
Definitions of community   4
'Need' and concepts in care   6
The restructuring of communities   10
Ideology   14
Social policy   18
Community care, providers and users   19
Structure of the book   22

2 A history of community care   **26**
Introduction   26
The role of the state and state intervention   27
Social care and the Industrial Revolution   29
Early twentieth century   31
The welfare state   36
Thatcherism and the receding of the welfare state   42
Conclusion   46

3 Health services and community care policy   **49**
Introduction   49

Health, demography and attitudes 50
Health reform and legislation in the 1980s and
    1990s 51
Ideology, the new managerialism and the NHS 54
Funding health care 58
Health care, collaboration and community care 61
Mental health, illness and attitudes: from institution
    to community 65
Comparative health care policies 71
Conclusion 74

4 Social services, community care and the market 76
Introduction 76
Models of care 77
The community care legislation 80
The restructuring of social services and local
    authorities 84
The purchaser:provider split in social services 87
The role of voluntary and independent sectors 89
The funding of social care 92
Community care plans 95
Care management 97
Changing organisations and social work pressures 101
Comparative social care developments 104
Conclusion 106

**PART II   USER GROUPS AND COMMUNITY
           CARE 109**

5 Elderly persons and community care 111
Introduction 111
Demographic trends and ageing 112
Ageing, ideology and discrimination 114
Health policy and older people 116
Social care, personal services and social policy 117
Community care polices and caring for older
    people 119
Community care, elderly people and financial
    difficulties 120

Empowerment, community care and elderly persons 124
Comparative policies and community care for
    elderly people 126
Conclusion 128

6 People with disabilities and community care 130
Introduction 130
Definition 131
Issues of disablism and discrimination 132
Physical impairment, mobility and community care 134
People with learning disabilities 136
Independent living, people with disabilities and
    community care 137
Disability, civil rights and collective organisation 140
Comparative policies for disabled persons 142
Conclusion 146

7 Mental health, homelessness and housing policies 148
Introduction 148
Mental health and homelessness 148
The role of housing policies and homelessness 150
Impacts of homelessness 152
Community care, housing provision and
    mental health 153
Hospital discharge, public safety and violence 154
User empowerment and disempowerment 157
Comparative policies in mental health and housing 159
Conclusion 162

8 Women and community care 164
Introduction 164
Women, caring ideology and the family 164
Women as all-round carers: informal and formal
    care 166
Women and community 169
Women, financial hardship and community care 170
Women, health and community care 172
Debates on the feminist critique of caring 173
Comparative policies 175
Conclusion 176

9   Minority ethnic groups and community care   **178**
Introduction   178
Racism and 'othering'   179
Racial discrimination and community care services   181
Family care and minority ethnic groups   183
The voluntary sector: charities and mixed provision   185
Comparative policies   189
Conclusion   190

10 Citizenship, participation and community care   **192**
Introduction   192
Citizenship and social democracy   193
Community care, user involvement and citizenship   194
Participation, power and empowerment in
      community care   197
Citizenship, community and communitarianism   199
Conclusion   202

11 Summary and Conclusions   **204**

Bibliography   *211*
Index   *237*

SERIES EDITOR'S PREFACE

In this volume Harry Cowen subjects the shift of policy from institutional to community care to rigorous and careful analysis. Starting from a historical base, he moves out to consider the implications of such a shift in both social policy areas and for user groups. Throughout the book, the author relates issues of community care to wider social policy concerns and to the role of ideology and political ideas in shaping the contemporary social policy agenda. This, then, is a project with a wide scope and it is hoped that readers will also find that it has depth as well as breadth. For me, the careful analysis of the relationship between current policy and social divisions is timely and welcome, as is the discussion which permeates the work on the way in which policy both impacts on social divisions and is, in part at least, shaped by them.

Other major cross-weaving and interlocking themes of the book may be said to be *marketisation* and *citizenship*. Part of Cowen's argument – and it is only part – is that the move towards the particular community care configuration we have has been influenced by:

- A governmental ideological preference for seeing the market as a more effective and more acceptable distributor of welfare goods than the state. The creation of managed or *quasi*-markets in health and in the personal social services is seen as shaping the nature and scope of policies in relation to community care.

- A reassessment of the relationship between citizenship and social policy. Here Cowen invites us to consider whether the marketised and consumerist emphasis of community care policy is a reflection of a shift away from an ideological orthodoxy that saw welfare needs as legitimately met as part of a citizen's social rights.

Cowen's analysis of these questions is supplemented by consideration of how longer-scale ideological positions – in relation to gender, social class and race – interact with these essentially *'new Conservative'* innovations to construct a policy agenda and a policy context for the care of often vulnerable groups of welfare state users. Given that one of these groups – the elderly – are not only with us but likely to be with us in greater numbers in the next millennium these are important considerations.

Michael Sullivan
Swansea
March 1998

PREFACE

Towards the end of the 1980s the Conservative Government un-
veiled the second tier of its massive social policy legislation
programme, in the form of government reviews, White Papers and
bills relating to community care. Lecturing on a social work course
at the time, it was no easy task to keep up with the new developments; evidently the pulse of policy change was quickening. Only
now, however, does it seem that we are in a reasonable position to
accurately assess the results of the strategy and legislation at the
closure of this decade. Undoubtedly the community care policy was
a major constituent of the social policy portfolio. Yet the government initially recoiled from making available to local authorities
the necessary 'start-up' resources. The three-year delay in fully
implementing the legislation was portentous. Community care was
to become one of social policy's most controversial areas, straddl-
ing two of T. H. Marshall's sacred pillars of the welfare state – the
health and social services.

It was problematic to gauge any tangible impacts of the legislation with only partial implementation during the early years.
Academic commentaries were far from plentiful, although the
weekly 'Community Care' continued to keep practitioners well informed. April 1993, the effective date for full implementation of
the NHS and Community Care Act, was considered by many to be
the start of the new market-based community care. In this respect,
community care policy is in its infancy, compared with housing
policy, although in other respects it stretches back a long way. As
the second half of the decade has progressed, academic assessments have appeared in plenty, usually on particular aspects of
community care. As we shall see, community care policy reflects so
many different elements as to necessitate constant vigilance in

keeping abreast of developments. This will continue to be the case as the new Labour Government's social policy programme takes shape. Having said this, it becomes all the more important to adopt an overview of community care policy; one must weave together disparate strands for the purposes of policy evaluation at the macro level. Community care policy must be approached philosophically, socially and politically, given that the manner in which a society cares for its communities reflects how it views its citizens *per se*.

Hence, the book is not simply factual, in the sense of describing relevant legislation and directives; it deals with the underlying political assumptions which, it is argued, account for defined pathways of change. The book expressly engages in locating ideological perspectives and the basic interconnections between state strategy and community care policy. Accordingly, it does not specify guidance on how to implement good practice; rather it aims at articulating and explaining key issues in community care policy: for instance, the impact of comprehensive restructuring and real cutbacks in socal expenditure upon users and employees; the human ramifications of a major policy redirection from institutional to home-based care; the appropriateness of quasi-market mechanisms for determining the delivery of care; the ascendancy of managerialism and the heightened profile of the independent sector. At the same time, it seeks to make comparisons with social policy and community care practices in other cognate economies.

The text sets out to communicate with two prime audiences: undergraduate/postgraduate social policy students, and practitioners. Neither category is monolithic. Students from the professions such as health, social work and housing may find the contents useful. Specialist practitioners as well as managers and policy makers operating at a strategic level may also find the book of interest. It is not intended to create an unreal division between theory and practice or between practice and policy. Students need to know about practical matters; by the same token, practitioners should be appraised of the wider policy environment, the historical roots of policies and available explanations for social problems.

As already implied, the book does not strive to engage with every constituent or cognate area of community care: for example health visiting, community health nursing, occupational health or community drug services. Already a discrete body of literature exists in community care, much of it concentrating on a specific client group, such as older people, people with physical disabilities, people with learning difficulties (formerly termed 'mental handicap') or people with mental health problems. A separate specialist literature on the medical and nursing functions of community care is obtainable; other specialist tracts deal with issues of the client assessment process or offer useful case studies of community care plans and local authority implementation. The reader should also be aware that this book does not address issues of provision for children, which are related to local authorities' statutory responsibilities under the Children Act 1989 and subsequent legislation.

Research is developing on the themes of empowerment and participation. This particular work does not attempt to replace such literature; instead, it aims largely at synthesis. New insights and material are presented, for instance with respect to managerialist ideology and community care, and developments in the Jewish community. For those who wish to pursue individual topics in greater depth, the reader will encounter suggestions for further reading at the end of each chapter, and a comprehensive bibliography at the back of the book. A conceptual and historical framework is constructed for understanding the changing direction of community care. Hence the reader will come across the term 'paradigm', meaning a generally accepted concept, theory or idea dominating an epoch. One cannot but be impressed by the contrast in the 'spirit of the age' as between the 1946–1978 years of the classic welfare state and the 1979–1997 period of new right (or neoliberal) Conservatism, a distinction manifested in social policy legislation, not least for community care.

The volume is divided into two fundamental parts, the first dealing with overall structural and institutional reforms, while the second examines specific user groups. In one sense, the parts are integral; in another sense, each section raises a discrete set of distinctive issues demanding close and separate scrutiny. Material is drawn mainly from the contemporary book literature, journal articles, magazines and newspaper commentaries, plus certain primary interviews.

ACKNOWLEDGEMENTS

I have received various forms of encouragement and assistance during the writing of this book, and welcome the opportunity to offer the following acknowledgements. First, thanks are due to departmental colleagues for general encouragement and generous assistance with references and for helping out with the delicate juggling of my teaching timetable. Second, I am grateful to Guy Daly for critical commentary on Chapters 3 and 10 and acting as 'sounding board'; to Dee Carter for comments on Chapters 6 and 8; to Mike Littledyke for technical aid in compiling charts, and Jim Keane for insights into the insurance industry. Appreciation is also due to David Owen, of Warwick University, for help with source material on minority ethnic groups. I wish to acknowledge the kind cooperation of the Manchester Federation of Jewish Social Services, and in particular Janet Blumenthal and Mark Cunningham, student social worker (for access to material from his DipSW project); the Merseyside Jewish Welfare Council, and specifically Suzanne Green, Lorraine Coleman and Sue Stansfield, student social worker; the Gloucestershire Chinese Women's Guild, and especially Mew Ning Chan-Edmead. Early encouragement and guidance from Mike Sullivan, and Christina Wipf Perry of Prentice Hall Europe, proved most valuable. Likewise, comments from the anonymous academic readers have greatly improved the text. Of course, I take responsibility for any possible lingering shortcomings. Last, but not least, I wish to acknowledge the support and facilities made available by the Department of Community and Social Studies, Cheltenham & Gloucester College of Higher Education.

PART I

SOCIAL POLICIES IN HEALTH AND SOCIAL CARE

1
INTRODUCTION: COMMUNITY, POLICY AND IDEOLOGY

Prime focus of the book

Community care in social policy is dual-edged, not least because of its ambivalence as a concept. Approaches towards it have changed historically, according to their ideological underpinnings, that is, the predominating social values and institutional frameworks of the time. Currently, the issue of community care is high on the social and political agenda of UK and other governments. Indeed, with the ceding of certain public sector activities such as community care provision to the private and independent sectors it has become effectively a means for running down the welfare state. Government community care legislation has refashioned the contours of health and social care provision since the 1980s. Hence, the resultant changes demand close analysis not simply in the legalistic sense, but in order to assess the impacts upon a range of social groups.

This book argues that community care policy must be understood critically and historically. Community care policy is not only about shifting structures and frameworks, but about the specific client groups such as elderly people, disabled people, people with learning difficulties, and people suffering from mental distress, all regularly marginalised from mainstream social policy. They have been socially 'othered' and often trapped by poverty. Policies in this respect have both reflected and affected the othering of social groups, a process encompassing social class, gender, age and ethnic discrimination.

3

At the same time, the policy shifts have also exerted consider-able impacts on the people employed in the health and social care services responsible for the delivery of community care, and expected to respond rapidly in a swiftly changing institutional environment. It is important to comprehend the nature of these organisational shifts, their ideological redirection and reappli-cations of technology, but also their short-term and long-term consequences. This is an area which cannot be treated in a tech-nicist manner; how a society cares for its communities reflects how it views its citizens.

This introductory chapter attempts to shed light on the defini-tive issues in community and caring. It shows how historical eco-nomic and social changes impinge upon both community and caring; it identifies the key providers of community care and the key issues concerning the recipients of community care.

Definitions of community

As suggested, the term community care is ambivalent. The term 'community' alone is the subject of a multiplicity of texts in such discplines as political philosophy, anthropology, geography and sociology (for example, Weber, 1958; Frankenberg, 1969; Bell and Newby, 1971; Plant, 1974; Willmott, 1986; Anderson, 1991; Crow and Allan, 1994). Much of the debate here turns on whether com-munity is a geographically based concept, essentially relating to neighbourhood, or whether it is a purely relational notion con-cerned with the ways in which humans communicate with each other more generally. But community is a value and not just a factual description (Plant, 1974; Skidmore, 1994). It reflects ideo-logical assumptions as to what is considered good or bad. Its meaning may be historical, cultural, personal or political. Bornat (1993) illustrates the breadth of the concept in collective life (e.g., Willmott and Young, 1957; Cornwell, 1984; Bryan *et al.*, 1985; Cain and Yuval-Davis, 1990).

Raymond Williams, a major social and political theorist, fre-quently engaged with community in seminal works such as *Culture and Society* (1958) and *The Long Revolution* (1965). His *Keywords* (1983) traces the evolving meanings of community from 'local' in the nineteenth century to 'community politics' of the twentieth century when community, juxtaposed to the more middle-class notion of 'service' to the community, has been used as an organisational tool for direct action. Whatever the definition, suggests Williams, the word is never used in a pejorative sense or viewed unfavourably – a plausible explanation as to why the term 'community care' has been adopted by all shades of government as part of their social policy.

But one may also readily understand how the meaning has retained for many a romanticised aspect reinforced by the perspective that community is a feature of the past which has now yielded to the fragmentary thinking and relationships of post-modern developments or the regressive journey from social relationships of community to those of casual association (Tonnies, 1955). Nevertheless, more contemporary 'oral history' studies on neighbourhood (Bornat, 1993) have called into question such romantic ideas conveyed by the 'rural' and 'urban working class' community studies (Willmott and Young, 1957; Jackson, 1968; Dennis *et al.*, 1969; Frankenberg, 1969).

Bulmer (1987) suggests that in spite of the multiplicity of meanings, two elements remain crucial to the definition of community from within a social care context: first, the focus upon local social relations within a geographical area; and second, the sense of belonging which is also entailed in the concept. However, the one is not necessarily entailed within the other. To be part of a geographical neighbourhood does not mean being part of a community or strong social network, namely, because of the factors of inclusion and exclusion. With the 'universal' economic and social changes of the late nineteenth and twentieth centuries, the physical boundaries of community have been increasingly displaced by the symbolic boundaries marking insiders from outsiders (Cohen, 1985). Such insider–outsider distinctions, argue Crow and Allan (1994), are increasingly significant, especially in relation to ethnicity in modern British society.

This issue of community and the growth of symbolic boundaries is important in community care. Black and Asian people are among clients in need of 'community care' (Chapter 9). So too are the other 'official' clients of community care such as disabled people (Chapter 6) and people suffering from chronic mental illness (Chapter 7), 'exiled' into the large psychiatric institutions from their social network and forced 'to negotiate membership of a new network and (become) institutionalised' (Skidmore, 1994, p. 38).

It is worth reminding ourselves that in recent history the ideological 'othering' of the physically different, the weak, the disabled bodied and mentally impaired led to the ultimate fate of genocide under Nazi social policy – part of the latter's project in delineating the unnatural from the natural (Cowen, 1994). Many of these groups still encounter social hostility and remain dependent upon being accepted into the formal network of community care.

'Need' and concepts in care

If we accept that there is a need to care, then it makes little sense discussing social policy outside the context of needs. But what do we mean by 'needs'? Can we define and measure them? Generally, there are two major approaches: one argues that basic, 'objective' needs exist; the other argues that needs can only be socially relative, that is, they depend on the culture or the specific society. For our purposes, the most significant and pertinent contemporary attempt to erect a universalistic framework belongs to Doyal and Gough (1984, 1991) who identify the basic, universal needs as good physical health and personal autonomy, differentiated from a discrete series of intermediate needs. They contend that all people have the right to a basic need-satisfaction. Such basic needs constitute the very preconditions for being able to participate in social life.

But what is an adequate *standard* of basic need-satisfaction? This will vary between cultures, so that *social* needs, which relate to issues like sickness and poverty, may arise from shared social conditions among certain social groups, and may only be dealt with at a social rather than an individual level. Clearly, social needs' definition is a socially contested one because of variation between societies (Bradshaw, 1977). Bradshaw notes that the concept of social need is inherent in the idea of social service, 'which historically has been organised to meet recognised needs' (ibid. p. 33). He erects a taxonomy of needs delineating normative need (defined by 'experts'); felt need (equating to want); expressed need (felt need transformed into action, i. e. the effective demand for a service); and comparative need (according to the characteristics of those receiving a service).

Hence, social needs and social policy inhabit a political territory. A critical literature bears testimony to the ways in which needs are subject to manipulation: privatisation policies, for instance, have shaped our ideas of autonomy (Lodziak, 1995). At an empirical level, the Leeds Metropolitan Pilot Study (Wetherly, 1996) provides a useful case in the political implications of need-satisfaction. First, there has to be a central role for the state or the public sector. Also, as implied by the Commission on Social Justice (Borrie, 1994), the meeting of social needs requires national strategies for social justice. Again, the legislative requirement for assessment of needs at the local level (NHS and Community Care Act 1990) demands resolute interagency collaboration – a persistent failing to date in community care. Furthermore, without the participation of local users, it is virtually impossible to acquire information on *unmet* needs (Wetherly, 1996).

As we shall see in Chapters 3 and 5, social policy leaves unmet for socially excluded groups the basic need of good physical health (Benzeval, 1997) and the autonomy necessary for participation in social life. The possession of autonomy presupposes education. Widening access to education is important for facilitating satisfaction and autonomous living. But for almost two decades governmental education policy was posited upon a model of individual choice which marginalises those still in need of the basic educational provision. (Because of this, the new Labour Government placed education at the top of its own social policy agenda.) With respect to provision for the intermediate need of appropriate health care, more than 400 empirical studies have documented the widening health divide in Britain between rich and poor from 1985 to 1993: yet the government policy response was minimal (Benzeval, 1997).

Another significant intermediate need wedded to basic health is for adequate protective housing. For instance, poor or costly heating will produce hypothermia among elderly people. As later chapters discuss, homelessness has risen, while the supply of social housing provision has been severely curtailed. Other policy areas relating to the meeting of intermediate health needs, as identified by Doyal and Gough, include adequate nutritional food and clean water, a non-hazardous work environment and a non-hazardous physical environment. Under the realm of 'autonomy', bearing closely upon mental health, the authors catalogue the intermediate need for security in childhood; significant primary relationships; physical security; economic security; education; safe birth and child bearing.

The notion of care also invites unpicking. Some would argue that it has no intrinsic connection with community and indeed leads us away from the idea of community altogether. To quote: '[The] affective bases of community care are kinship, religion and race, not community . . . Kinship remains the strongest basis of attachment and the most reliable basis of care that we have. This is especially true among women' (Abrams, cited in Bulmer, 1987) and is immediately apparent as soon as one realises that much of the care provided is of an informal nature; further, a fine dividing line runs between formal and informal care. Bulmer suggests four diverse sources of community care: statutory care, commercially provided care, voluntary care of the formal (and public) category and informal care which tends to be private.

What is the meaning of care? Bulmer (1987) points out that although the term seems self-explanatory, one is frequently unclear as to the types of help, support and protection in question when the term is used. There is a difference between the often demanding 'tending', entailing physical contact, and other non-physical material and psychological aspects of caring such as general support for elderly or frail persons or mentally distressed people, and more general expressions of concern. Thus care comprises physical tending, material and psychological support, and the more generalised concern with respect to others' welfare (Bulmer, 1987).

Clearly, until the public sector intervenes, the real care falls in the tending categories and within the informal and most personal context. And this is precisely where the issue of gender becomes central. Historically wives, women and daughters have usually borne the weight of care, providing an invisible form of labour and consistently deflecting the burden away from the state – a condition of exploitation which is compounded by community care policies (Dalley, 1996). On the other hand, when policy makers act on the assumption that women will automatically follow their culturally designated caring roles, they do so in a climate where males are often not acceptable as carers.

These overarching social assumptions of the feminine naturalness for doing the caring (as well as caring *about* the people close to them) and the unnaturalness of the male to do the caring (while nevertheless accepted as caring about another person) are inextricably linked to the fact that in defining care, its foundation has traditionally been viewed as the nuclear family: 'With woman as carer, man becomes the provider; the foundation of the nuclear family is laid . . . It becomes the ideal model to which all should approximate. Its basis is an ideological "familialism"' (Dalley, 1988, p. 15).

It will be argued in this book that community care policies are founded on this ideology of familialism. If one accepts the thesis that all policies are premised upon such an ideology, it calls into question the validity of the distinction often made in the literature between formal and informal care. Bulmer (1987) suggests a continuum between formal and informal care running across four diverse forms of care: statutory; commercially provided; voluntary; and informal care. A major aspect in the study and implementation of community care policies is the extent to which formal and informal care may be interwoven. Yet the idea of a continuum may also hide a rigidity and lack of flexibility. To quote Dalley (1988, pp. 115–16): 'concepts such as the continuum of care, which sees dependent people moving from one form of care into another as their dependency-related conditions improve or deteriorate, often fail to recognise the regimentation that that may involve.'

Since state policies, as we shall see, have been framed so as *not* to interfere with traditional family (private) patterns of caring, those in need of care, including aged people, and no longer capable of caring for themselves have become dependent upon family members (and upon women within the family in particular). When the family can no longer care for the person, the state has taken over almost total responsibility, rendering the client in turn totally dependent on the state institution, for example a mental hospital or a residential home (Bulmer, 1987). The caring relationship, in that it involves persons in forms of dependency to a lesser or greater degree, also implies the exertion of power and the empowerment of some people or groups over others.

Conversely, the dependants of care may all too easily become disempowered. It may be argued that many forms of dependency are socially constructed. At the same time, one cannot separate this personal and socially constructed dependency from economic circumstances and economic dependency. How far for instance have community policies empowered people with physical disabilities (see Chapter 6)?

Disempowerment and the concomitant loss of autonomy has been inviolably associated with institutional care by many critics and commentators who (as we shall discuss in Chapter 2) strongly advocated for social policy the deindustrialisation of care, especially from the large mental asylums – the archetypal 'total institution' (Goffman, 1961). But with the advent of deinstitutionalisation as policy, the question is raised as to whether this has empowered the newly deinstitutionalised users of services. Community care policies of the 1990s are indeed premised on deinstitutionalisation as a panacea for a host of problems.

To summarise, it is important to differentiate types of care in assessing the gendered nature of caring and where burdens fall. Familialism is in this respect an ideology which underpins official community care policy, implying an effective continuity between informal and formal care. The condition of dependence experienced by those in need of care rests on personal circumstances, social relationships and state ideology, and bears upon their potential to exert control over their own lives. Many influences have affected the communities and the relationships of care, not least those of economic restructuring.

The restructuring of communities

As we have discussed, neither 'community' nor caring relationships should be viewed in a static manner; similarly, we need to study policies in the context of change. We will examine the factors of change which have affected the restructuring of communities, and the impacts of change upon the lives of community residents.

In the first place, economic conditions and economic change in capitalism invariably affect the parameters of community by shaping the life chances of residents, not only individuals but whole social groups. Economic restructuring has been globally significant over the latter part of the twentieth century (Abercrombie *et al.*, 1994). Multinational corporation activities affect the fortunes of most local areas. Disinvestment decisions endanger local citizens' financial protection against impending sickness, infirmity and uncertain family support. Intensifed international competition and rapidly shifting technologies have radically reshaped the fortunes of working-class areas where high unemployment has tranformed older industrial communities, although perhaps surprisingly the impacts have not been entirely negative due to the continuity of informal social networks (Harris, 1987; Morris and Irwin, 1992). A highly influential explanation of restructuring is post-Fordism.

Post-Fordism

What is post-Fordism? Lipietz (1988) suggests that since the early 1980s, with the movement away from mass production techniques in the manufacturing of goods (as with Ford cars), a radical change has occurred in the method of capital accumulation, towards immediate flexibility in production methods, financial systems, marketing strategies and organising labour. Such developments have led to a greatly increased mobility and the globalisation of consumption patterns. In the process, unemployment and part-time working has grown, accompanied by personal uncertainty, insecurities and the diminished ability of collectivist organisations (trade unions) to effectively counter the forces of capital. Correspondingly, a fundamental restructuring of state interventionism has taken place, replacing the Keynesian philosophy of full employment goals and economic demand regulation.

While not fully rejecting this rather economistic theory, Jessop (1994) views it as flawed as applied to Britain, whose economy resembles more of a 'Schumpeterian workfare state' than a classical post-Fordist model. On the other hand, more direct critiques question whether the radical governmental changes in contemporary capitalism are explicable solely in terms of post-Fordist economic restructuring. Can the theory be applied to welfare services? Pickvance (1991) claims that public service provision in Britain has lacked sufficiently robust structures to facilitate participation at the local level, while Bagguley (1994) argues that post-Fordist forms of restructuring vary according to particular sectors and geographical areas. He suggests that the interpretation of welfare state developments as post-Fordist is too functionalist and economy-focused. Nevertheless, one may detect in welfare provision such post-Fordist *tendencies* as market power, deinstitutionalisation processes, community care, the growth of contracting and subcontracting, and managerialism. But such tendencies, claims Bagguley, are subject to the outcome of social struggles, which are not allowed for in post-Fordist theory.

Again, we may view the series of British reforms such as contracting and the invasion of the public sector by market relationships as particular local responses to global post-Fordism. In this vein, Pierson (1994) questions whether the reforms allied to post-Fordism have necessarily promoted the flexibility claimed: extending consumer choice to some will restrict choice for others. The problem of adopting post-Fordism as a total explanation of new directions in welfare policy is that it underrates the significance of the political dynamics behind policy, aside from other factors which may completely fail to optimise flexibility.

Post-Fordism, then, too easily detracts from the role of social response and disssent in the formulation of social policy. An unquestioning equation of welfare with manufacturing is unhelpful. But when combined with an analysis of the ideological and policy dimensions of marketisation and managerialism, post-Fordist theory does help us to understand the new paradigm of social welfare policies, and the impacts on the social care workforce (discussed in Chapter 4).

Anyway, rapid economic change cannot be divorced from cultural change. Modern advanced capitalist societies evince regular movement of residence or location, the compulsion to purchase consumer goods, and current shifts in the pattern of political allegiances. Permanence as a social experience yields to immediacy, ambivalence and a sense of restlessness labelled the post-modernist experience (Berman, 1983; Lash and Urry, 1987; Cooke, 1990). Flux and unpredictability provide the unlikely environment for caring which demands maximium continuity and a sense of stability. As we shall see in Chapter 5, the fact that more people than ever are living to a much greater age, needing care and attention raises a number of cardinal issues, not least the facility for contemporary communities to care in such a period of ephemeral values.

These economic and cultural changes are deeply ideological. A seminal shift in British social and economic life at the end of the twentieth century is the move from a general quasi-collectivist approach, where institutions and organisations directly supply welfare and caring services, to a model based on individualism and essentially competitive market relations. This has meant an increasing reliance on private enterprise for formal caring activities during the 1980s and 1990s. Again, individualistic thinking in the territory of everyday life pervades informal care and the chances of consistent support for the society's vulnerable groups of people (to wit, the inauspicious rise in the numbers of homeless people and the related lack of access to health and social services (see Chapter 7)).

Policy and related political changes profoundly affect urban and rural communities. Such policies are not confined to community care policy but they produce direct impacts in that respect. Transport policies and cognate economic areal regeneration strategies affect a local population's geographical mobility. Urban planning and rehousing policies, like the postwar British new towns' programmes and the docklands' regeneration schemes have refashioned, reinvigorated or destroyed existing communities. But such policies may result in all kinds of intended and unintended consequences affecting different social classes, gender and minority ethnic groups. The Housing Act 1980, enforcing the mass sale of council housing, deeply implicated the fabric of local communities and the life chances of various social groups. Welfare and social policy, including social security and health and social care policies, affect the economic and social stability of local groups. The community care legislation of recent decades considerably affects social relationships and caring; it also starkly reflects the overall ideological shift in Britain's political climate at the turn of the 1980s when New Right inspired perspectives and policy prescriptions came to replace a general consensus on social democratic approaches to the welfare state (discussed more fully in Chapter 2). White Papers on health and community policy and the NHS and Community Care Act 1990, along with such related legislation on the structure of local government, are principal markers for the direction of British social policy at the century's end.

To recap on those factors affecting the restructuring of communities, global and local economic and technological change destabilises financial security for family care and limits institutional provision. Attendant cultural factors mean rapid geographical and political mobility and new social allegiances in an epoch when more elderly people require care based on the old family structures. Ideological reorientation away from social democratic collectivism towards private enterprise values means circumscribed access for many potential users. Finally, community outcomes are not only contingent on community care policies but on the equally fundamental transport, local government planning and social security policies. In the next section we consider the particular meaning and importance of ideology in community care.

Ideology

Eagleton (1991) suggests that there are now so many meanings to 'ideology' as to render the word useless. The *Oxford English Dictionary* speaks of visionary speculation, adapted by Skidmore (1994, p. xii) as 'speculation' for *creating* an ideology for community care. Eagleton's extensive definitional list nevertheless makes it clear that ideology connotes the exercise of power and the socially dominant mainstream ideas which shape the paradigms of state policy. Such sets of ideas or beliefs are more than political party tags – they reflect ways of understanding and social relationships (Plant, 1974). Ideology informs 'community' and 'policy'. Hence, the scrutiny of policy is a historical investigation of ideological change and shifting power relationships, and the ideologies of welfare which only became dominant in the second half of the twentieth century.

A sea change in 'thinking and acting' occurred during the 1980s and 1990s, resulting in the overthrow of communism as a political system in 1989. One may basically describe the shift as the wholesale move from collectivist to individualist modes of thinking, interpreting and responding: a turn away from the 'holistic' mass scale solutions to nuanced, discrete answers to social problems. Social theorists and philosophers have interpreted this social redirection as a replacement of the 'modern' paradigm by post-modernism. This has effected a turn from collectivism to individualistic thinking, and from common forms of identity to pluralistic expressions of difference. In the world of economic production it has entailed moving from Fordist mass production methods to the post-Fordist customised operation and the adoption of a 'flexibility' in labour markets where jobs are no longer certain. In the political sphere, consumerism, whereby citizens express their citizenship through market choice, has replaced the politics of citizenship (Lash and Urry, 1987; Harvey, 1989).

14

The new political mode of seeing the world elides the economic and the political. Criteria for decision making on welfare have been subject to power of the market place for most of the century's final decades, tempered by forms of mixed welfare.

The market and quasi-markets

The use of markets in the provision of care services represents an essential ingredient in the paradigmatic policy shift over the past twenty-five years. Privatisation formed a key plank in the 1979–97 Conservative Government's social policy strategy for reducing political state intervention in the British economy. Its sustained privatisation programme encompassed the selling of nationalised industries and local authority council housing. Furthermore, the practice of contracting out to commercial or non-profit organisations was adopted by public sector institutions as crucial to the operation of health and personal social services, giving high priority to the independent sector (voluntary and private organisations).

The idea of the market as the regulator of all relationships in society stems from Adam Smith's classic *Wealth of Nations*; it is the nub of the respective academic justifications by Friedrich Hayek (1962) and Milton Friedman (Friedman and Friedman, 1962) of the New Right's project to 'roll back the state'. However, the incursion of the market process into the public sector does not reflect a 'pure' classical market. This commercial welfare provision by the state has been termed 'quasi-market' as a way of distinguishing it from the pure market model (Le Grand, 1990). Such a mode of allocating resources is most likely to remain during the new Labour Government's period of office.

Whereas it is argued that 'marketisation' of public services benefits consumer needs and preferences by pushing down cost levels, quasi-markets nevertheless prioritise the private profit principle over the concept of public service. In the process, they tend to exclude social groups by dint of cost considerations. Although commercial operators may not strictly make a profit, financial criteria as opposed to the prioritising of service will nevertheless drive their activities so as to remain in business. In the event, only certain consumers are able to meet their price. Acquisition of requisite skills for managing budgets is time consuming, and seems appropriate for the training of professional groups such as medical staff. Additional resources and skills are needed within quasi-markets which the state welfare services do not as a rule offer. All this suggests that quasi-market provision may well prove more *expensive*. (The issue of quasi-markets in health and social care is discussed in Chapters 3 and 4.)

Nevertheless, the market model survives into the new millennium despite the waning of New Right influences in British party politics. As we shall see in Chapter 2, the major postwar ideological developments from collectivism and Fabianism to New Right anti-statism transfigured the social policy agenda. While the 1990s have edged towards a more comforting ethical communitarianism and a growing concern with social justice, the Thatcherite paradigm is in a sense partly 'irreversible' (Barker, 1997; Gray, 1997).

Such overarching ideological change is accompanied by a new language of managerialism, which one may view as the late twentieth century's reassertion of technicism and positivism. The new managerialism, particularly marked in policy, invokes revised measurements of worth and the attribution of a different 'value', displacing the traditional organisational philosophies in the whole policy arena. Concepts of 'efficiency', 'effectiveness', 'quality assurance' and 'competence' offer new criteria for decision making on resource allocation (Farnham and Horton, 1993; Clarke *et al.*, 1994; Clarke and Newman, 1997) (see Chapter 4).

Managerialism

We need to understand managerialism as a manifest ideological feature of social policy and the public sector. It is possible to locate two key features characterising the new role of management within the public sector. First, managerialism highlights the inspirational, charismatic elements of senior managers in enthusing the wider workforce to commit themselves to their respective organisations. The second focuses on the devolution of responsibility, conveying enhanced status for local management in 'downsized' organisational settings, which 'requires a closeness to and interaction with customers' (Clarke *et al.*, 1994, p. 3).

New managerialism's fundamental role in the restructuring of the public sector should not be underestimated. It links the network of markets and partnerships to the recomposition of the labour force and the current emphasis on customers, and simultaneously connects the two worlds of business and the public sector. Furthermore, it redefines power relationships in the social policy sphere in two ways. The redefinition of relations with users, clients and citizens, for example, tends to undermine previous models of social welfare where professionals 'represented' their clients' interests. Now managers are deemed to act as the definers of customer 'needs' and 'demands'. Thus the public sector workforce is redefined, mainly due to managerialism's challenge to traditional assumptions of professionalism. To quote Clarke *et al.* (1994, p. 6): 'The old professions are weakened by a meta-narrative which is at the same time able to incorporate and undermine them.'

This may mean on the one hand an increase in opportunities, such as for professional women. Yet on the other hand, given the large numbers of women concentrated in the 'caring' professions, opportunities for women may contract. Considering their heavy recruitment from the private sector, managers are undoubtedly playing a crucial part in the organisational transformation of the public sector. Business representation on public sector management boards has grown. Public sector management programmes are now integral to the public sector, while the reorientation of an organisation's professionals into management positions is a widespread feature of the devolution and decentralisation of management systems. In all cases, both managed and managers operate within the discourse of a new managerialism.

But another way in which ideology bears upon social policy and community care lies in the construction of value attached to specific social groups. Patriarchal societies subjugate the social value of females to male domination; British imperialism located black peoples as biologically and 'thus' naturally inferior to whites; Nazism cast Jews and mentally disturbed people into the category of subspecies; in Western societies old people's low status correlates with their low economic productivity. In the context of community care, the influences of such ideologies continue – witness the cases of ageism (Chapter 5), disablism (Chapter 6), sexism (Chapter 8) and racism (Chapter 9). Every 'othered' group has been subjected to ideological processes of exclusionism that inevitably limit possible inclusion in the 'community' and entitlement to rights of citizenship (Chapter 10).

Social policy

The definition of social policy is closely tied to the postwar welfare state (Bulmer *et al.*, 1989). Social policy, representing the wider framework for decision making in community care, is usually made by government or the state for promoting individual welfare, and clearly affects the distribution of resources among various social groups. Its strict meaning is not unproblematic. 'Policy' is formulated by the state, through a set of state institutions and personnel, and has authority (Weber, 1946). More specifically, social policy is interpreted as a field of study involving the economic, political and sociological analysis of how 'central and local governmental policies affect the lives of individuals and communities' (Jary and Jary, 1995, p. 617). The focus in this discipline of social policy has tended to be 'who receives what?' between groups in society. Given its genesis during a period in which the welfare state represented an assertion of working-class rights along socialist principles, the literature has historically reflected social class divisions (Hill, 1996).

But social policy is itself socially constructed; definitions of social policy have altered with the dominant structures and ideologies in western capitalism (Cahill, 1994; Sampson and South, 1996). Such a reconstruction is part of the global pattern of economic and social transformations (see Chapters 2, 3 and 4). With the expanding social policy environment, the parameters of the subject have widened, from the tightly constrained study of social administration (largely a functionalist approach, scarcely concerning itself with underlying philosophical and ideological assumptions), in traditional areas of social security, health and personal social services. A more critical perspective emerged from the 1970s which addresses issues of need, citizenship and empowerment. Interest has grown more recently in the comparative dimensions of social policy, while the economic is considered integral to social policy analysis (Bulmer *et al.*, 1989; Jary and Jary, 1995; Hill, 1996). The focus on inequalities currently embraces gender and policy, reflected in the rapidly expanding feminist social policy literature (Maclean and Groves, 1991; Dalley, 1996; Pascall, 1997; Ungerson, 1997; also see Chapter 8 of this book). Such refocusing is an element of the more general widening of social scientific inquiry; other inequalities between social groups, for instance 'old old' as against 'young', single parent females and disabled people, now cut across class divisions. All these categories figure prominently in Townsend's seminal schema of poverty in the United Kingdom (Townsend, 1979) which simultaneously captures the profile of community care user groups.

Social policy today covers a range of topics such as social security, education, housing, health, personal social services, employment, comparative analysis and community care. A number of these are closely related in their operation and impact (although not necessarily treated so by policy makers). Thus, in-depth analysis of community care must connect with cognate social policy sectors. Similarly, evaluation of impacts in community care needs to engage with new social divisions and with economic and philosophical reconstructions of social policy – not least, with the redefining of welfare state functions and the enhanced profile of 'welfare mix' strategies (Drover and Kerans, 1993).

Community care, providers and users

In this section we will describe briefly the deliverers and the recipients of community care. The deliverers may be roughly divided into those employed by the health and social services, those working in the voluntary and independent sectors, and the informal carers. It should become clear that the types of personnel involved have changed along with the transformations in institutional policies and frameworks. These changes will be charted in some detail in Chapters 3 and 4. One should also note that the boundaries between health service and social service providers converge at many instances, but still lead to policy and practical conflicts. New responsibilities are placed upon local authorities for fronting services such as mental health largely through their financial control over community care budgets. Yet much controversy surrounds the precise loci of responsibility, delineation of roles and agencies of control. Collaboration and the precise duties of community health professionals are major policy implementation issues. But problems of collaboration and designation of responsibilities are compounded by the new practice of a purchaser:provider split, itself a method for fostering market relationships within the public sector.

The independent private sector is largely responsible for running the majority of residential and nursing care homes and contracting for various social care services. Voluntary services play an enhanced role in the development of domiciliary services, but they are closely tied to the guidance and financial resourcing of the local authorities (a situation which has caused apprehensiveness among voluntary organisations and community groups over loss of autonomy – as discussed in Chapter 4). Judging from government community care policy statements, the housing department's role is less obvious. Housing authorities, housing departments and housing associations participate in strategic collaboration for providing housing appropriate to community care (see Chapter 7).

The role of care workers and the social services (Chapter 4) has been fundamentally overhauled under new legislation, so that new structures for community care management in local authorities require different functions and responsibilities for certain social workers, many of whom have become community care locality managers. Emphasis is now on management as opposed to special professional expertise. But the role of social services personnel formerly paramount in the area of residential care is reduced dramatically with the involvement of the private and independent sector.

Organisational restructuring has not simply changed the roles of many workers in the social services, but has transformed their working conditions. The purchaser:provider split has sundered the social worker role and thus reduced the orbit of discretion and autonomy; the increased emphasis on accountability has produced frustration and resentment in having to place 'organisational' demands before client needs. Because the central state's financial support has not met the radical changes required, insecurity and fear of redundancy is now part of the social care service climate, and the displacement of professional staff by a semi-skilled and unskilled workforce (Hadley and Clough, 1996). One associated result is the rise of stress levels among social services employees (Chapter 4).

Informal carers usually come from within the structure of the family, and are key providers of community care, not only in Britain but in most comparable societies. A controversial topic of debate is the extent to which government policy is prepared to direct resources in supporting informal care, as well as the ideological debate as to whether informal care frequently provided by females should be completely formalised.

But what about the *recipients* of community care? In the strictly functional sense, these have tended to be elderly persons, physically disabled persons, mentally handicapped persons (or people with learning difficulties) and mentally distressed people. Collectively, elderly persons have become important recipients of care during the last few decades as their numbers have grown in relation to the younger groups in the population. Unlike physically or mentally disabled people with a biological impairment, old people 'grow into' the need for care as their physical or mental faculties decline. It is this imbalance between elderly people and other demographic groups that has caused the biggest ripples in the policy pool, given the cost implications of a growing non-employed, non-tax paying section of the population in receipt of services and the fact that very old people require residential and nursing home care. Further issues concern social ageism, whereby older people are deemed no longer 'useful' to the society beyond a certain age, victims of a socially structured dependence (Chapter 5).

Since World War II, government policies have attempted to integrate people with impairments into the community. However, disabled persons have traditionally received little formal assistance; it is argued that this is essentially due to the continuation of an institutional discrimination against disabled people that still lies at the root of modern welfare organisations (Oliver, 1990; Barnes, 1994). Disabled people face barriers of 'othering' and myth, so that an impairment becomes socially transformed into 'non-able', a process hastened in the health service by the predominance of the medical model which focuses entirely upon the impairment.

People with learning difficulties (formerly termed mentally handicapped) in particular form a group of people frequently 'othered', marginalised on the edges of society as abnormal or deviant. The 'normalisation' perspective held by 'progressive' theorists and practitioners is that mentally handicapped persons have a 'right' of integration into family and the community 'as normal'. But the aim for normalisation is not an unproblematic, non-ideological issue; it begs the question of 'the norm' and uncritical acceptance of formal social goals (Ryan and Thomas, 1987).

People suffering from poor mental health or severe mental distress comprise a user group which has received perhaps most policy attention during the post-World War II period, yet it may be argued that it is a group currently subjected to the most neglect from current community care policies. The quality of service delivered to this group is at the heart of pubic controversy over the dramatic shifts from institutional to community care. As the numbers of patients in long-stay hospitals have declined and the large urban mental hospitals have closed, mentally distressed people have attracted extensive media attention mainly where unsupported community 'care' has resulted in violence or death (Chapter 7).

Although minority ethnic groups do not form functionally distinct community care user groups, they nevertheless meet a set of related problems arising out of arguably discriminatory practices and procedures which demand special attention, for example in the sphere of mental health service provision. While new legislation on community care was heralded as promising benefits for minority ethnic groups at the start of the 1990s, it seems no longer clear that the expected benefits are actually forthcoming.

To sum up, health and social care services are the statutory institutions for delivering care, although the issues of collaboration and delineation of responsibilities come to the fore with the changing functions of the respective authorities. New legislation has enhanced the role of the independent and voluntary sectors in the mixed economy of care. Restructured institutions have led to re-defined roles, work location and revised responsibilities for health and social workers with the emphasis on managers as opposed to professional specialists. Informal carers remain the dominant and essentially female group of unpaid care workers, and hence vulnerable to oppressive and exploitative policies.

Structure of the book

We have charted a territory of definitions, problems and issues; the remainder of the book will be structured in such a way as to present the reader with the historical, political and functional dimensions of community care policy provision in Part I, and particular issues regarding user groups in Part II.

Part I, 'Social policies in health and social care', comprises three chapters embracing changes in community care. Chapter 2 traces the history of community care and the changing ideological role of the state in its relationships with individuals, groups and civil society. It considers the significance of political theoretical perspectives, and surveys the different approaches to care in the Victorian era, the twentieth century, and the years of the 'fully fledged' welfare state followed by the period of a 'receding' welfare state during the 1980s and the 1990s, sustained by a powerful consumerist social philosophy.

Chapter 3 focuses on health services in community care, and identifies specific issues and problems in health care provision. It assesses the particular significance for community care of the health reforms and related policy statements, the importance of the new quasi-markets, and the influence within the new structures of managerialism and the purchaser:provider distinction. The chapter analyses the social construction of health and attitudes towards health and sickness, the ideological significance of policy debates over deinstitutionalisation, and normalisation and mental health treatment. Comparisons are made with the experiences of other economies.

Chapter 4 deals with social services at the social care end of community care and the impacts of the market on the traditional social service structures. Attention is paid to the new relationships developed between community care purchasers and the independent and voluntary sectors. The chapter identifes specific issues surrounding community care planning and care management, and the impacts of the new managerialism upon the social work profession and the caring profession cultures in general. Again, the chapter concludes with an assessment of social and community care developments in other countries.

Part II of the book, 'User groups and community care', comprises six chapters engaging with problems facing discrete user groups. Chapter 5 concerns itself with elderly persons and community care and the particular social constructions placed upon the ageing process, analysing the uncertain 'individualised' futures of elderly people, and evaluating the implications of demographic trends and the interrelationship between class, gender and policy, comparing Britain's community care policies for elderly persons with those in other countries.

Chapter 6 highlights the situation of disabled persons and community care, and the ideological and social barriers faced by this user group. The chapter studies the tensions between the philosophy of 'independent living' and community care plans, and evaluates the feminist critique in respect of caring strategies; it examines government resistance to legislative change, the importance of more recent employment legislation, and developments of a new social movement in other comparable economies.

Chapter 7 takes a further look at the issue of people suffering from mental distress, primarily relating to issues of homelessness, housing and community care. It explores pertinent housing strategies against a background of declining public expenditure, and the ramifications of discharge strategies for both public safety and patients' rights. The chapter also considers matters of service user involvement and policies abroad.

Chapter 8 discusses the position of females and community care and the dual roles women play in the community care process. It examines the coordinates of the care–family–female nexus and state social policy, and the feminist critiques which have demonstrated the political significance of the personal domain.

Chapter 9 deals with the position of minority ethnic groups in relation to community care, and with understanding the connections between racism and health and community policies. The chapter investigates the implications of minority ethnic group family structures for policy, and the underlying ideological assumptions of white British decision makers. It considers practices and issues of community care in specific minority ethnic communities, and looks at how other societies are handling discriminatory practices.

Chapter 10 focuses upon the idea of citizenship in relation to community care, and considers debates between liberalism and communitarianism, and of participation and decision making regarding the new contractual relationships. It examines the interrelationship of citizenship, empowerment, participation and accountability with respect to community policy, community care goals and marginalised social groups.

Finally, Chapter 11 offers an overview of Part I and Part II of the book, and arrives at a set of conclusions regarding the outcomes of community care policy during the 1990s and speculations on future directions.

Further reading

CLARKE, J. and NEWMAN, J. (1997) *The Managerial State: Power, politics and ideology*, London: Sage. Locates the key elements of managerialist ideology in the public sector.

LAVALETTE, M. and PRATT, A. (eds) (1997) *Social Policy: A conceptual and theoretical introduction*, London: Sage. A useful textbook on concepts, theories and trends in social policy.

HOGGETT, P. (ed.) (1997) *Contested Communities: Experiences, struggles, policies*, Bristol: Policy Press. Issues of identity, government and participation.

LEONARD, P. (1997) *Postmodern Welfare: Reconstructing an emancipatory project*, London: Sage. A critical theoretical analysis of the shift in the social welfare policy paradigm.

ALCOCK, P., ERSKINE, A., and MAY, M. (1997) (eds) *The Student's Companion to Social Policy*, Oxford: Blackwell. A valuable new reader written by leading social policy commentators.

2
A HISTORY OF COMMUNITY CARE

Introduction

Community care, as noted in the introductory chapter, is an ambiguous concept. It must be grasped historically; policies pertaining to community care may formally reach back to the mid-twentieth century, but policies relating to community care also boast a longer historical life, concerned with the care of marginalised and disabled groups. Indeed, the term's origins are somewhat hazy, with general references by the Local Government Board to 'more homely accommodation' than the workhouse, and to an overt community care policy in 1946 (Walker, 1982). Yet the issues and policies for the discrete groups emerge much earlier, in a broader context of 'social policy'; such issues need closer examination.

The changes in contemporary social policy must also be understood in terms of key economic changes and changing perspectives in the marginalisation of particular social groups, and the potential conflicts which constitute an intrinsic part of the political and economic debate between free market laissez-faire ideas, advocacy and state intervention.

In this chapter we will analyse the role of the state and the issues of state intervention as they have sustained themselves ideologically since the nineteenth century, the impacts of the industrial revolution and the particular features of social care provision of the Victorian era under social paternalism, the 'interwar' period of the twentieth century, the development of collectivist ideas and the significance of the period of World War II, the archetypal collectivist period of the postwar welfare state and the initiation of community care policy, and finally, the importance of the period from 1979 to 1997, a period in which much social policy has been rewritten, not least in the area of community care.

The role of the state and state intervention

At the centre of social care issues lie ideological tensions over caring responsibilities for those unable to care for themselves: a space between individualism and the state. Such tensions have been reflected in the contending political perspectives on the state which have driven the social policy agenda: liberalism, socialism, Fabianist collectivism and theories of the New Right.

Liberalism

'[At] the heart of liberal politics is a strict distinction between the state and civil society', suggests Bellamy (1993, p. 27). However, there are different kinds of liberalism, and even the liberalism of the nineteenth century may be divided into the utilitarianism of Jeremy Bentham and the liberalism of J. S. Mill. Bentham argued that, '[it] is the greatest happiness of the greater number that is the measure of right and wrong' (*Fragment of Government*, 1776). The only justification for state involvement in individual affairs was if it brought pleasure. The emphasis fell on interference to ensure that more individuals enjoyed the free pursuit of such.

Mill was more evidently engaged with the adverse consequences of capitalism's unharnessed individualism upon more vulnerable people, and the ills stemming from untrammelled capitalism. The solution to social problems was to provide institutions ensuring that a net benefit was gained, expressed as the number of people receiving their services. Mill pointed to the severe limits of laissez-faire practice where it marginalises collective responsibility for those who need care.

Fabianism

Fabian collectivism was in the socialist tradition, but unlike Marxism it aimed at socialist reform and gradualness, taken as inevitable given the continuing growth in the size of the state sector in modern societies (Bellamy, 1993). This was also interpreted by the Webbs and economic historian R. H. Tawney as a move towards collectivism and equality and away from inidvidualism. Their advocacy of powerful social and economic regulation of the state and the inauguration of huge public service institutions was crucial in influencing the progress of the British Labour Party and the development of the twentieth-century welfare state, besides its major infuence on the growth of social work. Tawney (1931) argues strongly in favour of the moral strengths of solidarity, community and equality (Lee and Raban, 1988; Wright, 1993).

Neo-liberalism and the New Right

The collectivist 'consensus' behind the building of the welfare state, especially during the mid-twentieth-century period, has been vociferously challenged by the influential ideology of the New Right. One can trace the roots of the latter back to the market liberalism of the early nineteenth century and the ideas of the political economist Adam Smith. Confusingly, the New Right is also a part of the panoply of *conservative* politics and government in Britain and the United States of America since the late 1970s. The New Right's prime attack was upon the state's high profile in the areas of social provision. Economists Friedrich Hayek and Milton Friedman espoused the superiority of the market system of service allocation as against any form of state planning and high levels of public expenditure. Notions of the mixed economy or a middle way between capitalism and socialism are rejected as naive. State welfare encourages dependency, while welfare measures are responsible for the creation of a permanently unemployed 'underclass', a rather suspect thesis which eliminates other causes of unemployment (O'Sullivan, 1993).

To summarise, late nineteenth-century liberalism reflects the uneasiness of educated advocates of industrial capitalism in search of the limits to laissez-faire principles, recognising state intervention as a prerequisite for protection of marginalised groups in need of care. Fabian collectivism, on the other hand, was more positive in promoting public service institutions on a major scale, an overt collectivism espousing equality and social reform which was to provide the ideological underpinnings to the classic welfare state. The third ideological stream of political economy market principles represents a rejection of social welfarism and has dominated politics at the latter end of the current century.

Social care and the Industrial Revolution

The rapid rise of industrial capitalism in the nineteenth century brought in its wake the first large-scale social institutions, accompanying the dramatic growth in the size of urban populations and settlements engendered by the industrial revolution. Social problems could no longer be exclusively 'individualised'. However much the ideology of laissez-faire was promoted with respect to economic behaviour, governments increasingly intervened in making provision for the many groups unable to fend for themselves.

The Industrial Revolution

During the first half of the nineteenth century, the factors of rising population, increased urbanisation and large-scale production forged an industrialism which, in turn, heralded the beginnings of public health, the rise of the workhouse and a series of attempts to deal with disability and mental illness. Edwin Chadwick, a social reformer much influenced by Bentham, worked to minimise the burden of people upon the public purse. A Poor Law Board was instituted to oversee the 1834 Poor Law Amendment Act, while workhouses were set up for mainly able-bodied people. These were capitalist institutions of transparent social control. With the official segregation, disabled people were confined to the family or to the special institution; disability became a shameful condition – a stigma (Oliver, 1990).

The workhouses proved to be a dumping ground for aged long-term sick and mentally distressed people. No asylums were built for them but they were quite simply shut away in the workhouses along with elderly and chronically sick people. However, the classified 'lunatics' were quickly viewed as too problematic. Social reformers called for regenerated asylums, agitation which led to the Lunacy Act of 1845 establishing the institution of county asylums, and a Lunacy Commission for regulating all asylums and public, private and voluntary hospitals catering for lunatics (Murphy, 1991).

Although the asylums were another form of social control of

dangerous groups, they have been praised for the undoubted commitment of their initiators engaged in 'a serious attempt to manage a growing social problem in an enlightened way and those who founded them genuinely hoped that sufferers would benefit' (Murphy, 1991, p. 35). But it became cheaper to commit 'lunatics' to the asylum instead of the workhouse and the concept of 'treatment' for mentally ill people soon receded (Murphy, 1991).

Chadwick's social reforming and substantial attention to sanitation engineering and municipal initiatives also guided the early years of public health. The Public Health Act 1848 coupled with the Medical Act 1858 (establishing a General Council for Medical Education and Registration) represented 'perhaps the most dramatic interference into the everyday life of its citizens that the state had thus far envisaged' (Midwinter, 1994, p. 55) – 'a grudging statism' by which '[gradually] various groups were officially exempted from the full rigours of self-help . . . But for the rest, and even for some of those in need, Victorians hoped that private philanthropy would render the necessary temporary palliatives' (Fraser, 1973, p. 114).

Towards state collectivism

During the latter part of the nineteenth century, collectivism developed according to the principles of J. S. Mill's increasing stress upon community responsibilities as opposed to individual liberties. At the same time, electoral reform extended suffrage, the labour movement's power grew but so did the more conservative ideals of philanthropy and social commitment. Modernisation of local government at the closing years of the century meant that the increasing number of public initiatives could be more effectively implemented; municipalisation familiarised the public with notions of collective provision.

This period of 'piecemeal collectivism' (Midwinter, 1994), which stretches to World War II, is important due to the intensified use of the 'institution' rather than 'individual' initiative as a solution to social problems. But such 'knee-jerk' institutionalisation came under sustained attack from sociologist Erving Goffman (1961) and social policy analyst Peter Townsend (1962), both highly influential advocates of deinstitutionalisation.

The archetypal giant hospitals spawned by the charities and the poor law legislation were built between 1870 and 1940. They provided 113,000 beds in Britain by 1891, and the numbers had more than doubled at the start of World War II. The drive towards improved public health was transformed into the notion of public housing; the new local authorities were given powers to demolish unsanitary housing and to rehouse inhabitants as it became clearer that the private sector could not deal with the problem (Midwinter, 1994). Old people still suffered from a dire lack of provision, with no effective pensions.

Finally, an important element of social care in the nineteenth century, destined to play a consistent role in the next century, was voluntary assistance and charities – part of the philanthropic tradition. The number of charities aimed mainly at 'moral reform' of the poor greatly expanded in the late nineteenth century, charting the way for the social services of the current century. The Fabian view was that voluntary agencies and the state should possess parallel spheres of influence and that voluntary action was innovative and significant. Later such boundaries were to blur.

Social care, then, during the high point of the Industrial Revolution was delivered in the context of a rising population and burgeoning urbanisation. The period was marked by the rise of the workhouse, which became the dumping ground for mentally distressed, old and chronically sick people, an efficient method of hiding them from the public gaze. Similarly, the introduction of the huge asylums reflects the belief in the institutionalisation of the 'social problem', a feature of this epoch of social reform and administrative intervention. The opening of the twentieth century prefigures the turn to state collectivism and a developing concern with community responsibilities. Public health raised its profile, and public housing entered the political agenda but the voluntary sector remained an important source of welfare provision.

Early twentieth century

The beginnings of the twentieth century with respect to social care represented a continuity from the late Victorian era, with the frequent implementation of social policies in the state sector, albeit on a piecemeal basis. On the whole, as we shall see, groups in need of care have remained marginalised.

The early period of the twentieth century in Britain was shaped by a liberalism prepared to countenance socialist ideas on the basis of the duties and effectiveness of public bodies in the deployment of society's collective force 'to mitigate the worst effects of a capitalist system, to intervene within but not to overturn a capitalist society' (Fraser, 1973, p. 132). Socialism with a Fabian face and the rise of the social reformist investigators such as Charles Booth became increasingly important, especially in counteracting the ravages of the Poor Law (the individualistic ethic was still powerful).

The voluntary tradition enjoyed a high profile in the domain of state policy over this period. Lloyd George's budget of 1914 embraced an unprecedented number of grants to voluntary organisations in the social care field (Brenton, 1985). Although one interpretation was that the voluntary tradition was being phased out by growing statutory provision, it was also argued that public subsidy would enable voluntary agencies to survive and offer them a permanent role in relation to the statutory sector. Their role for elderly people was enhanced in the later National Assistance Act 1948.

The late implementation of old age pensions during the 1905–14 Liberal Government's period of strong health and educational reform reflected recognition of the dire needs of old people as a group. Consensus behind the old age legislation may be understood in the context of continued pressure for state pensions through the late nineteenth century (including Booth's findings that the incidence of poverty was largely due to old age). More and more provision for workers in uncertain conditions was diverted from the province of the Poor Law (Fraser, 1973).

With World War I the liberal spirit suffered an irreversible defeat – the death of liberal England (Dangerfield, 1936) opening up a rift in perspectives on the future of politics, economics and social policy. Nevertheless, an essential continuity survived in the economic and social conditions and in the impulse towards social reform (Midwinter, 1994).

Recession and the interwar years

The facts of war if anything placed state intervention higher on the political agenda than it had ever been, nurturing 'the growth of a strong collectivist urge' (Fraser, 1973, p. 164). Unemployment, health, housing and education became the four key items in social policy's postwar reconstruction. But of course, with the growth of worldwide recession, unemployment was the central problem irresolvable by private charity or the vagaries of the Poor Law. State national insurance was introduced as an antidote to poverty (but throughout the 1930s many people's employment benefits were cut). The founding of the 1934 Unemployed Assistance Board introduced a national level of assistance benefits replacing the previous local discretionary system.

However, the realms of social policy scarcely provided for disabled persons, who were more or less permanently 'in the community'. (Barnes (1994) points out that no real development has occurred in disabled persons' benefits since before World War II.) One encounters in the 1920s and 1930s a reinforcement of the nineteenth-century ideological legitimation of the oppression of disabled persons with the continuation of Social Darwinist 'survival of the fittest' ideas in support of Galton's eugenics both in the USA and Britain. In the former, 25,000 people were sterilised so as to prevent them passing on their 'feeble-mindedness' or their criminality to succeeding generations (Jones, 1993, p. 9). People with learning difficulties were kept separate from others in such a climate (Ryan and Thomas, 1987). Public enquiries and professional accounts in mental health testified to the horrifying conditions in local asylums, such as the 1920 Ministry of Health inquiry into conditions at Prestwich Hospital in North Manchester. Testimony revealed a disquieting lack of especially trained staff, patients not allowed out of the building, poorly dressed patients and poor monotonous food (Jones *et al.*, 1975). Government ordered a Royal Commission on Lunacy and Mental Disorder, set up in 1924 in response to the 'reckless' claims that 'large numbers of sane persons were being detained as insane, that the whole system of human administration was wrong, and that widespread cruelty existed in our public hospitals' (cited in Jones *et al.*, 1975, p. 237). The Commission's findings expressed concern at the lack of community care once the mental hospital discharged anybody. Jones (1975) observes that a preoccupation with aftercare (plus pre-care and research) consistently figured in reports throughout the 1920s and 1930s; gradual change took place inside the mental hospitals, but the stigma of mental treatment certification endured. 'The seeds of the community care idea were well established by 1930' and anticipating the dissolution of the asylum system (Murphy, 1991).

With respect to elderly persons, old age pension legislation continued, although welfare policy concentrated more on poverty among those of working age. The numerous old people began to dominate the workhouse. The Conservative Government passed the Widows', Orphans' and Old Age Contributory Pensions Act in 1925 partly in 'response' to long-term labour movement pressure from 'an increasingly restless' postwar working class, given the problems of facing old age, and partly due to the Chancellor of the Exchequer's aim to offer some balance to his tax concessions for industry (Thane, 1996). This introduced contributory pensions as a means of eliminating old age pauperism.

Beveridge's *Insurance for All and Everything* had proposed an all-in insurance plan embracing unemployment, health, dependants, disability and widows' pensions and a lowering of the pensionable age for working men to 65. The Labour Government's Pensions Act 1929 extended pensions to 55-year-old widows; the 1937 Pensions Act advanced pension rights to certain groups of independent workers on a voluntary contributions basis. Take-up was low, however. Despite the considerable efforts to care for the country's old people during the interwar years the governmental programme was not really successful in guaranteeing economic independence to elderly people. Numbers on Poor Law relief grew by roughly 5 per cent per annum. Gilbert (1970) notes that elderly people were representing an increasingly larger proportion of those obliged to seek public charity. Furthermore, attitudes towards the care of old people developed in a similar fashion as those towards the care of unemployed people throughout the 1920s and 1930s. It was not until the beginning of World War II, with the institution of supplemental pensions, that the notion of meeting need drew official acceptance.

The newly styled 'public health hospitals' arising from the Local Government Act 1929 offered no real medical service for old people, who were simply classified as 'chronically sick'. At the same time, an elderly entrant to a workhouse (now termed Public Assistance Institutions) would lose pension entitlement. Conditions remained sparse and socially restrictive (Means and Smith, 1994). Indeed, the 1929 Act exerted a profound effect upon elderly people, who were often displaced from medical wards (McEwan and Laverty, 1949, cited in Means and Smith, 1994).

The Fabian style of state collectivist solutions to social policy problems was encapsulated in the 'reluctant collectivism' (George and Wilding, 1994) of the economist John Maynard Keynes, whose *General Theory of Interest, Money and Employment* in 1936 was a plea for full state intervention to achieve full employment, characterising the spirit of comprehensive state responsibility for people's social lives: the solution to unemployment was more, not less, public expenditure.

World War II and the significance of Beveridge

The years of World War II were important for social policy as a bridge between the interwar years and the period of major implementation of a welfare state in Britain from 1945. Early statements, plans and policies provided the foundations of welfare statism, although wartime social policy reflected the 'emergency' psychology of the period. Private, voluntary and local authority hospitals were swiftly and arbitrarily merged. State intervention in industry was strong. Many mental institutions were taken over for military personnel; the most disturbed patients were restricted to a few wards (Jones, 1994). The intentions were nevertheless good. 'Certainly, the chronic sick, the disabled and the infirm elderly came very low down on the list of priorities', yet 'there was a desire to plan for a better society when the war was over, and the wartime Coalition Government was aware of it' (ibid. p. 125).

The crucial marker for statist social policy in these years was the 1942 Beveridge Report, which constructed the framework of the coming 'Welfare State' around the five social problem 'giants': 'Want', 'Disease', 'Ignorance', 'Squalor' and 'Idleness'. For removing want, the state social security plan was to offer benefits as of right, with the individual 'topping up', a philosophical fusion of community and individual responsibilities. Full employment was the nub of the Beveridge scheme; *Full Employment in a Free Society* (1944) mirrored Keynes' advocacy of total state intervention for full employment. The comprehensive insurance in benefits, embracing sickness, unemployment, disability, workmen's compensation, old-age, widows' and orphans' pensions, funeral grants, and maternity, ran from 'cradle to the grave' (Fraser, 1973; Stevenson, 1984; Jones, 1994). Commentators have remarked upon the social consensus forged by the Beveridge Report. Elizabeth Wilson (1977) and subsequent feminist writers, however, have examined the implications for women of Beveridge's underlying assumptions, which included women's 'rightful' place as being in the home. As we shall see in Chapters 5 and 8, women, as 'family' and the community's 'carers', as well as 'patients' have suffered financially, physically and psychologically from the implementation of such assumptions.

To recap, the period was dominated by the problems of economic development and the political importance of the rise of socialism. In response to the latter, the Liberal Government's social reforms planted the seeds of welfarism. Voluntary bodies maintained their significance. The inception of state pensions reflected the alarm at the widespread poverty among old people. Economic recession dominated policy making and sharpened the recognition for state interventionism, but it was still a low period for disabled and mentally disturbed groups, whose conditions were atrocious. Attention given by the health authorities to aftercare was closely tied to voluntary sector activity, an early anticipation of community care policy. Nevertheless, it proved an era in which institutionalisation predominated, the workhouses were packed with old people, and the extension of pensions scarcely signalled their humane treatment. Finally, the period is notable for setting the ideological climate which governed the years to follow. Keynesian theory plus the onset of world war sharpened the profile of state interventionism, while the Beveridge plan paved the way for implementation of the classic postwar welfare state and the simultaneous marginalisation of women in the private spheres of 'caring'.

The welfare state

The years from 1945 to the late 1970s constitute the epochal welfare state even though, as we have seen, there is a continuity from the preceding period and across World War II. The social democratic political model flourished – a new ideological paradigm for the provision of state services.

The welfare state and ideology

Although its full strength is debatable, government consensus over the idea of substantial state intervention transformed the state into a mixed economy and introduced state intervention in social welfare (Sullivan, 1994). The welfare state's response to Beveridge's five giant problems in the social sphere represented the latest stage in a negotiated tension between individual and society. Economically, it assimilated the Keynesian thesis that full employment was only possible with strong state intervention and economic planning (Shonfield, 1969; Fraser, 1973; Lowe, 1993; Deakin, 1994).

The social democratic ideological framework of the welfare state, while initially dominated by the socialism of the Labour Party, was broadly adopted by subsequent Conservative governments (Sullivan, 1994). The landmarks became the three pillars of the Welfare State: the Education Act 1944; the NHS Act 1946 and the National Insurance Act 1946 (Rees, 1985; Timmins, 1996). Yet considerable evidence testifies to the deep ideological divisions remaining between the major political parties (despite the technical convergences over policy) and which resurfaced with a vengeance at the end of the 1970s (Lowe, 1993; Sullivan, 1994; Deakin, 1994; Timmins, 1996). Without an awareness of these undercurrents it is difficult to completely appreciate the ferocity of the attack upon the welfarist foundations of community care at a later period (Chapters 3 and 4).

The NHS and health care

The NHS Act 1946 (implemented 1948) was a social revolutionary measure even in the context of the evolving state provision of health services. Emerging from a Fabian tradition, it was nevertheless unprecedented in its free universalism (free at the point of delivery), a unique example of the collectivist provision of health care in a market society (Klein, 1995). The Act set up new regional health structures independent of local government, and although soon to develop growing pains, it became a beacon of British social life, with its family GPs and dentists, 'free' subsidised prescriptions and hospital services (Midwinter, 1994). Through the following decades, this more or less comprehensive state intervention in health care, a mix of state intervention and mixed funding was not a major source of ideological friction between the political parties (Sullivan, 1994).

The development of personal social services

The prior development of the personal social services was scarcely comparable with the health care services in that the term covers those 'residual' services provided for groups such as physically handicapped people, elderly persons or mentally distressed people by local government services. Hence, they remained poorly funded long after the launch of the welfare state. Since they were financially wedded to local authorities they were fragmented and unable to exert political authority. Accordingly, their clients could not wield much influence, in stark contrast to the spirit of the new welfare state and the concept of social citizenship.

The National Assistance Act 1948 officially negated the Poor Law. Intended to promote welfare, it remained central to the care of elderly people for decades. Part III of the Act created 'residential accommodation for persons who by reason of age, infirmity or any other circumstances are in need of care and attention which is not otherwise available to them'. Local authorities were also empowered to provide non-residential services for disabled persons. But progess was slow. Residential care homes (both private and voluntary) were still accommodating only 4 per cent of older people by the 1970s (Jones, 1994; Midwinter, 1994).

A breakthrough in the provision of social services occurred in the relatively affluent 1960s: generic training was offered in social work; popular support for active citizenship and community care and new scientific discoveries resulted in dramatic increases in public expenditure on personal social services. The Seebohm Committee inspired the Local Authority Social Services Act 1968 which instituted large liberally funded social services departments aimed at uniting different professions (Lowe, 1993). As we shall observe in Chapters 3 and 4, such growth in resources was to be short-lived.

However, voluntary care and provision remained crucial even during this period, especially in the sphere of informal care provided on a vast scale, so refuting earlier prognostications that it would wither away. By the 1960s, Citizens Advice Bureaus (CABs), Samaritans, NSPCC, Age Concern, CPAG, the Disabled Income Group and Shelter were all considered worthy of realistic funding. Until the 1970s the essential form of non-statutory care was the voluntary or informal rather than the commercial organisation which was to become typical under the later market-driven Conservative Government policies of the 1980s and 1990s (Chapters 3 and 4).

The development of modern community care

Community care became an 'official' target for government in the 1960s. Two government health and community care plans proposed growth in the numbers of GPs, health visitors, district nurses, home helps, sheltered housing schemes and sheltered workshops, targeting elderly people, physically handicapped people, mentally distressed people, mothers and children (Jones, 1989). Pressures intensified for health service institutions to reduce their numbers, while local authorities were encouraged to expand their facilities (Jones, 1989; Barnes, 1994).

This government reorientation towards a community care perspective seemed to reflect the period of antagonism against institutionalisation, as expressed in the writings of Goffman (1961) and Townsend (1962). However, the deinstitutionalisation policy at the time was not without its critics, including Richard Titmuss, a major social policy academic, sceptical of the government statements' generality in the absence of commitment to supply the requisite resourcing, financing and training (Jones, 1989).

Mental health

The Royal Commission on Mental Illness and Mental Deficiency reported in 1959, making the first use of the phrase 'community care' (Barnes, 1994). The subsequent Mental Health Act 1959 heralded the final closure of the large mental hospitals; it brought in non-compulsory admissions for the bulk of patients, and tightened up on procedures for compulsory treatment and detention. As noted earlier, the 1963 'plan' made provision for a whole set of community-based services as an antidote to the institutionalisation of the large mental hospitals. A government decision cut back on the numbers of mental hospital beds by some 50 per cent in 1961. This proved a disastrous policy decision with long-term repercussions. By 1974, 'there were 60,000 fewer residents in large mental hospitals than . . . in 1954, but very few services existed in the community . . . in most cases these people simply "disappeared" from the official statistics since no one followed up their progress or knew anything about their fate' (Murphy, 1991, p. 60).

The Department of Health and Social Security published *Better Services for the Mentally Ill* in 1975, conceding that the 1963 plans had proved unsuccessful, with the rise of admission rates, the continuation of mental hospital accommodation, few definite closures and poor staffing levels. The primary care team was the new focus. However, whereas this concept may have been appropriate for physical sickness and physical disability, it did not work so well for people with mental health problems, many of whose links with community or family are tenuous, and who require specialist social work expertise and attention (Jones, 1989). Relations were tenuous between health authorities and social work services in some areas. With the Local Government Reorganisation Act 1974 and the expansion of social services departments, increased responsibilities for care of this group devolved on to the social workers (Chapters 3, 4 and 7).

People with learning difficulties

The Mental Health Act 1959 was also seen as the legal basis of community provision for people with learning difficulties, in that it expanded the definition to encompass 'mentally handicapped people'. Local government health departments based on hospitals were expected to deliver a variety of residential, day and family support services, the legislation strengthened safeguards and defined the role of the Mental Welfare Officer, as with mentally ill persons (Tyne, 1982).

Progress in the delivery of community services for people with learning difficulties was slow. Admissions remained high, as did the institutionalised population, largely due to the breakdown of family and community support, besides factors such as poor information for parents on the availability of services (Tyne, 1982). Conditions in the hospitals were controversially poor. *Better Services for the Mentally Handicapped* (1971), a governmental statement, argued against segregation, and for a 50 per cent reduction in hospital places by the beginning of the 1990s, a growth in day centres, hostels, group homes and flats, and fostering, funded by local authorities and developed with social work support. Current hospitals were to be upgraded and psychiatrists were to play a greater role.

The new Seebohm social work climate and the pragmatic approach of normalisation (see Chapter 3) as opposed to segregation constituted two particularly important background aspects of government policy (Ryan and Thomas, 1987; Jones, 1989). But an intrinsic dimension of the problems of community care for persons with learning disabilities was ideological – an 'attitudinal factor'. To quote: '[The] mentally handicapped rate a low priority in the eyes of the general public, and despite the repeated pressures of the voluntary organisations and the reformers, despite the good intentions of successive governments, the situation is slow to change' (Jones *et al.*, 1975, p. 185).

With respect to physical impairment, the Chronically Sick and Disabled Persons Act 1970, in tandem with the Local Authority Act 1970, incorporated the 1968 Seebohm recommendations, enforcing local authorities to gather data and information on the scale of problems for people with disabilities (Barnes, 1994; Midwinter, 1994). These scarcely constituted mammoth changes for physically disabled people. Yet it signalled movement in local authority and voluntary agency perspectives, and in public attitudes and practice *per se*. But the Act and the cash payments were inadequately funded, a situation evoking widespread anger. Without proper funds, a number of local authorities 'made do' with sample surveys, despite the urgency for proper care of physically disabled people after years of neglect (Lowe, 1993; Midwinter, 1994).

Elderly people

Ostensibly, the reorganisation of local authorities and the expansion of social services after 1971 resulted in greater attention being paid to elderly persons by social workers. Local authorities were obliged to offer a greater variety of domiciliary care. Seventeen home helps and 15,250 meals per annum were available to every 1,000 people over the age of 75 by 1975 (Evandrou *et al.*, 1990), reflecting a general increase in national standards of care for elderly people because of the establishment of the new social services departments. This growth reflects the epoch of relatively high spending on social services, on resources and staff at the zenith of the British modern welfare state. By the 1981 Census, the numbers working in public administration, health and education constituted a massive one-third of the total workforce compared to one-tenth in 1881. At the same time, 175,000 full-time equivalent staff worked in personal social services, comprising 25,000 social workers, 50,000 residential care workers, 8,000 day care workers,

6,000 probation and aftercare officers and 13,000 worked in the voluntary and charities sector by the commencement of the 1980s (Midwinter, 1994, p. 119). Such trends were accompanied by creeping uncertainties and criticism of the welfare state, not least due to its perceived growing burdens upon taxpayers.

The classic twentieth-century welfare state, in sum, may be conceived as both structure and philosophy of the mixed economy and state interventionism that survived within a consensus masking deep political divisions which emerged later. The NHS was the marker of a universalist welfare perspective. By contrast, social services, formally responsible for marginalised user groups, remained poorly financed – a negation of welfare state ideology. But the dramatic changes of the 1960s, the startling expansion of social services and the increased financial support tendered to pressure groups give some indication of the era's material affluence and the close proximity between economic and social policies. Orientation towards a community care philosophy reflected the mounting opposition to institutionalisation of services. Yet while mental hospitals began to close, community services did not automatically replace them; problems of coordination surfaced between health authorities and social services. Although community provision now covered 'mentally handicapped people', few changes of substance were made. Public attitudes reviled attempts to remove segregation in the hospitals. By the same token, local authority initiatives received slight financial support. Finally, elderly people did benefit from improvements in standards of service by dint of higher levels of spending in the 1960s and the earlier 1970s.

Thatcherism and the receding of the welfare state

Although the summits of the welfare state discussed in the previous section represented an unparalleled standard of living and general levels of collective provision which in areas such as the NHS showed the way for other nations, escalating problems and associated criticisms eventually led to a set of policies based on individualism: the ideological antithesis of state welfarism.

Rising criticisms of the welfare state

The 1970s turned out to be a decade of quickening challenge to the welfare state, arguably stemming in the first instance from Marxist critiques consistently questioning the legitimacy of the capitalist state, followed by the ultimately more devastating attack from the political right and the consequent return of a Conservative Government to office at the end of the decade. The welfare state came under heavy ideological, political and popular attack. Recurrent crises of neo-Keynesian economic policies, the crises in industrial production of the Callaghan Labour Government, and the initiation of planned major cutbacks in public sector borrowing and expenditure culminated in the 1979 'winter of discontent' and the electoral defeat of the Labour Government (Lowe, 1993; Deakin, 1994; Sullivan, 1994).

The new Thatcher Government marked the unequivocal break with the welfarist consensus at the turn of the 1980s, a decade in which a whole set of different operating principles emerged. Intellectuals of the British New Right, led by Conservative Minister Sir Keith Joseph, directly confronted welfarist philosophy in the political arena with the market precepts of Hayek and Friedman, and argued that the welfare state was inefficient, ineffective, socially damaging, promoted conditions of dependency and eroded individual responsibility (George and Wilding, 1994).

The new politics of policy

The New Right replaced welfarism with a resurfacing of the 'natural order' based upon individualism and the tenets of the liberal economic market place. The new individualist agenda, even for caring activities, comprised a check list of activities which transformed community care: the inculcation of entrepreneurialism and managerialism, the privatisation of formerly public sector activities, commitment to the rule of law and the 'rolling back of the welfare state' to a residual rather than a mainstream position, the emphasis of the family unit as opposed to the state in caring, and finally, the positive promotion of inequality in creating a value framework which perceives inequality as both desirable and natural (Johnson, 1990; Hewitt, 1992; George and Miller, 1994; Lavalette and Pratt, 1997).

Social policy change under the New Right

The key changes deriving from the New Right perspective happened in the areas of social security, health and housing and local government. They tended to be least drastic in social security, given that 75 per cent of households derived part of their income from this source. However, the Social Security Act 1986 withdrew available money by 50 per cent, introduced Income Support, and replaced grants by loans in an attempt to reduce public sector social expenditure.

Structural changes in the NHS and government directives heralded the new managerialist philosophy of competition, pricing and privatisation of services in the early 1980s. Seminal reports, including Griffiths' *Report of the NHS Management Inquiry* (1983) for health and community care reforms lay at the heart of the new ideological turn. The 1990 Act removed prime responsibility from the NHS for people with mental health problems, physically disabled people, people with learning difficulties, and incapacitated old persons requiring long-term care (Jones, 1994). The direct impact of these policies for community care is studied in greater detail in the following two chapters.

Housing legislation in the1980s transformed the situation of shelter provision in Britain. The Housing Act 1980 offering the 'right to buy' to council tenants produced a huge growth in home ownership and a corresponding decline in public housing tenure (Forrest and Murie, 1991; Johnson, 1990; Midwinter, 1994). As we shall see in Chapter 7, while this redirection in property ownership was welcomed by many, the negative consequences have been far-reaching for 'vulnerable' groups. In terms of service provision, the later White Paper on 'Housing' (1987) and the Local Government and Housing Act 1990 proved to be as revolutionary. The strategy restructured local authority housing departments from being housing providers to housing enablers and further marginalised the council housing sector (Johnson, 1990; Cole and Furbey, 1994).

Community care and the 1980s

Given the host of changes in the health service and local government, the 1980s was a decade for developing the revised model of community care policy. This particular policy area, inextricably linked to heath care reforms, was subjected to a regular barrage of commissions, policy statements, White Papers and the final 1990 legislation infused with the New Right's ideology of management enterprise, financial expediency and markets.

The DHSS *Care in the Community* 1981 document outlined possibilities for shifting hospital patients out into the community. *Making a Reality of Community Care*, produced by the Audit Commission (1986), targeted the return to the community of elderly persons, people with learning difficulties and people with mental health problems. Later commissioned reports were steeped in economistic and managerialist rationale. As we shall see, the restructuring of health and social service organisations according to 'purchaser and provider' contractual market relationships has redefined the whole activity of social and community care.

Community care and the 1990s

Although the Act was passed in 1990, implementation of the majority of its contents was delayed until 1993 due to the lack of resources provided by the government, but also because of the local authorities' organisational and procedural lack of preparedness (Means and Smith, 1994). Walker (1993) suggests that the panoply of policy initiatives outlined above have meant for the current decade a residualising of social services through the deliberate fragmentation of community care, reflected in the purchaser: provider split, the systematic engagement of the market and a combination of decentralised services constrained by ever tightening centralised government financial control.

Although it was argued at the time that John Major's Government of the 1990s anticipated a departure from Thatcherism and the domination of New Right principles, the actual course of events suggests otherwise (see Chapters 3 and 4). Certainly the legislation effected a restructuring of social services organisation and a recasting of required professional skills, but also placed a different emphasis upon users as individual consumers with citizens' rights.

Finally, the restructuring of these services may be placed in the much broader context of a post-Fordist or post-modernist restructuring of capitalist economies in the late twentieth century, stressing flexibility, devolution of responsibilities and consumerist-orientated organisation fronted by general managers. One may argue that the effect of corporate restructuring on local government services and the welfare state as a whole has been incisive (Cochrane, 1994), although the theory that post-Fordist restructuring is universal and highly successful has not gone unchallenged (see Chapter 1) when measured against its real failures in promoting efficiency (Pierson, 1994; Warde, 1994).

The Thatcherite period, then, proved seminal by dint of the welfare state's receding significance. Political persuasions of both left and right mounted sustained critiques of its goals and operational outcomes, but the New Right gained more practical advantage from its market-based attack on the basic premises of welfarism and the 'nanny state'. The overall social policy agenda was overtaken by the new politics of individualism and entrepreneurialism, reinforced somewhat inconsistently by a moral familialism. Social policy changes shadowed New Right ideology almost step by step as social expenditure growth slowed down. Much of the groundwork for community care policy was accomplished in the 1980s, founded upon theories of economic efficiency and managerialist ideology. Formal implementation of the policy was slow during the 1990s because of the evident lack of initial seed funding for the local authorities; the repercussions for formal structures, user–provider relationships and the role of the state sector are nevertheless enormous.

Conclusion

To conclude, it is vital to situate community care in a historical context so as to understand clearly the ideological underpinnings of policy. Liberalism, socialist or social democratic collectivism and contemporary neo-liberalism represent polarities which at certain historical moments have shaped strategies in health and social care and the treatment of specific user groups. It is also clear that many current policies are not merely responses to contemporary problems, but also echo those formulated in a previous century to deal with rapidly growing populations and with the appearance of diverse groups experiencing physical and psychological difficulties. Proposed solutions in each case have posed problems of administrative efficiency, financial expediency and social control. For a long period the mass institution has reflected the growing state recognition of its 'community' responsibility, but the voluntary charitable tradition remains powerful. Whether state provision or the voluntary sector is pre-eminent, what is evident is that the institutional social policy framework has treated user groups more as burden than as citizens enjoying parity with the rest of society. Consequently, the early twentieth century may be seen as a sobering period in which user groups in health and social care were treated shabbily, more or less reflecting the social-class basis of industrial capitalism but also the deepening economic problems of the period. The close relationship between the poverty profile and the social status of these user groups is startling. The second half of the twentieth century marks a paradigmatic shift for social policy in the form of the classic welfare state founded upon a statist ideology. Social policy now meant collectivist rights and provision, yet the marginalised user groups were not truly recognised until the era of unparalleled economic affluence in the 1960s, which was a backcloth to the first explicit community care policies alongside the notable expansion in numbers of elderly people. While the first moves towards deinstitutionalisation signalled a revised form of community care, it was implemented much less fervently than later on. The Thatcher epoch seems equally as revolutionary as the welfare statism it challenged, informed by an overarching New Right economic and political ideology gaining in strength as economic recession deepened. Community care has figured highly in a new social policy agenda which has restructured housing, social security, the health services and social expenditure planning. In the next two chapters we shall examine the community care changes and their ideological significance in detail.

Further reading

Jones, K. (1994) *The Making of Social Policy in Britain: 1830–1990*, 2nd edn, London: Athlone. A concise historical survey.

Sullivan, M. (1996) *The Development of the British Welfare State*, Hemel Hempstead: Prentice Hall/Harvester Wheatsheaf. A clear account of state policies and welfarism in the postwar years.

Wilson, E. (1977) *Women And The Welfare State*, London: Tavistock. Still the classic critique of Beveridge's familialist ideology.

ROGERS, A. and PILGRIM, D. (1996) *Mental Health Policy in Britain: A critical introduction*, London: Macmillan. Lends an important historical dimension to the understanding of current policies.

JACK, A. (ed.) (1998) *Residential Versus Community Care: The role of institutions in welfare provision*, London: Macmillan. The institutional–deinstitutional debate by academics and practitioners.

3
HEALTH SERVICES AND COMMUNITY CARE POLICY

Introduction

Health care policy, it is argued in this chapter, is an essential ingredient of community care, but the policy decisions have been shackled by traditional organisational divisions between health and social care. Again, health policies reflect the ideological perspectives of government, and, in this respect, the substantial changes effected in health policy and administration during the 1980s and 1990s not only represent responses to demographic and social developments in the society, but also much broader ideological strategies in social policy *per se*, whereby collectivism gives way to individualism; public needs cede to managerialism and the market; and equity gives way to cost effectiveness and income generation. Yet such tendencies constitute part of the 'paradigm' shift occurring in a number of other countries where the burgeoning cost of health is posing a multitude of policy problems. The particular solutions being offered vary to an extent, but they are also clearly related to social and community care strategies – hence the great significance attached to the means for effective collaboration between health and social care agencies. In many cases, organisational cultures constitute the barrier; traditional professional hegemony and power are at stake, particularly between the medical profession and the allied 'caring' professions.

This chapter looks at the shifting attitudes to health and the issue of technological change, the specific health care reforms and legislation and their impact for community care, and the influence of new financing arrangements. Issues of the health–social care divide and collaboration difficulties in the context of community care are explored, as well as the mental health service–social care tensions and related ideological conflicts, and pertinent comparative developments in health care reform. Community care policies relating, in particular, to local authority social services form the subject of Chapter 4.

Health, demography and attitudes

Attitudes to health have been affected historically by economic and social conditions; they are also inextricably related to changing population profiles, technological developments and the ruling ideas on the causes and effects of health and sickness, such as organic explanations as opposed to environmentalism and holism. Demographic changes exert a profound effect on the demand for health services and upon their cost – especially at the younger and older ends of the life span (Meredith, 1995). The numbers of elderly, and especially very elderly, people are growing in most countries of the western world.

Demands for long-term care

This extended life span has led to a refocusing of health strategies. Chronic sickness is high among very elderly persons; their increased longevity brings in its wake a growing demand for long-term care, placing greater pressures upon health services. Ironically, the longevity with its concomitant pressures has been facilitated by the technological advances made in the medical sphere, developments which, in turn, tend to escalate health costs. It also raises the question as to *who* provides the long-term care, and *how* it will be funded – seminal questions at the centre of controversies in current community care (see Chapter 5).

One of the dangers of automatically linking increased longevity with cost is that it sets ageing and old people as a group in the mould of social burden, thereby contributing to the process of their 'othering' from society, that is, ageism. But whereas, as we shall see, the NHS and new health authorities are intent on offloading patients to the social care sector, the continuing hegemony of the medical professional staff strongly influences attitudes towards health and accepted modes of treatment, and the issues of jurisdiction over clients in the arena of community care. The tenacious hold on the acceptance of the 'medical model' reflects the power of the medical profession in defining the parameters of treatment in health policy; it has steered the medicalisation of health policies (Friedson, 1970; Cowen, 1994; Macdonald, 1995; Hill, 1996), not least in the United States, and is a prime reason for the tensions generated by the Conservative Government's community care changes, which clearly challenged the dominance of biomedical approaches to health. This is evident in the spheres of mental health policy, but also in the resistance of GPs to the governmental health and community care reforms.

Health reform and legislation in the 1980s and 1990s

Health services changed radically during the 1980s and 1990s, emanating from the government's ideological and political agenda. The thrust of the policies run along parallel lines with the reforms in social services, and must be understood in relation to community care legally incorporated under the NHS and Community Care Act 1990.

The 1983 Griffiths Report on the NHS

This first of the Griffiths Reports, on health services, was portentous in its advocacy of 'management' as the panacea for problems of service delivery, a style adopted for the social services and community care policy *per se* later in the decade. Sir Roy Griffiths, from the world of business and commerce, was commissioned by the government. He perceived the major problem as the absence of line management in the NHS. Despite resistance to this particular idea, the orientation towards general management was effected by a restructuring of a NHS which adopted the practices of managerialism and public sector resource budgeting.

Basically, all Regional Health Authorities, District Health Authorities and NHS hospitals were to appoint general managers for handling the foremost difficulty of the NHS – the absence of any evident line management hierarchy or direct accountability. A decentralised model went to the heart of the proposals. A NHS Supervisory Board was to be created, which the Secretary of State would chair, plus a NHS Management Board (which became the NHS Management Executive). In addition, clinicians were to be offered an enhanced involvement in management decisions. The speedily implemented report prescribed the ethos for the future. Imperatives and directives for greater efficiency were the new goals for Britain's health service provision.

The 1988 NHS Review

The NHS Review 1988 was the government's follow-up to the 1983 Griffiths Report, and the forerunner to the important White Paper 'Working For Patients' (1989). The Review was not a Commission but a clear-cut Cabinet tool for implementing Thatcherite policy changes in the organisation and management of the NHS (Holliday, 1992, 1996). The ideological driving force was the individualistic cast of New Right ideas, with various options for change advanced by the New Right's series of 'think tanks' such as the Adam Smith Institute (ASI), the Institute of Economic Affairs (IEA) and the Centre For Policy Studies (CPS). The resulting radical proposals embraced the adoption of an internal market, building upon the ideas of Alain Enthoven, an American health care economist, who also pioneered the purchaser:provider dichotomy created by the major legislation at the turn of the decade. Crucially, the 1988 Review initiated the division of the DHSS into a separate Department of Social Security and a Department of Health. This seems a curious act of policy in view of the major problems in health and social care collaboration for implementing the community care policies of the 1990s.

The 1989 White Paper 'Working For Patients'

The White Paper of 1989, born out of the 1988 Review, arguably represented the most drastic reform programme in NHS history and which confronted a host of long-standing problems, including differential standards of GP care, a failure in real responsiveness to consumers by the service providers, a concomitant lack of choice and clear variations in clinical practice between hospitals.

The White Paper outlined the following solutions:

- The separation of purchasing and providing, for stimulation of competition, that is, the creation of an internal market, directing health authorities to buy health services through negotiated contracts with self-governing hospitals, other health authorities and the private sector. At the same time, health authorities were empowered to 'market' their own services to other health authorities. The District Health Authorities (DHAs) were given the prime purchasing role.

- The creation of NHS Health Trusts, whereby hospitals and other NHS units were to become distinct self-determining trusts able to finance themselves through the marketing of their services. These NHS trusts became the main providers of care, unfettered by 'excessive consultation or supervision' (Mohan, 1995, p. 239).

- General practitioner practices initially with at least 11,000 patients (subsequently reduced to fewer than 7,000) were allowed to become 'fund-holding' practices. The Regional Health Authorities (RHAs) were to allocate funds to fund-holding practices sufficient to cover the costs of staffing and drugs, while the GPs were to contract for hospital treatment on their patients' behalf, and could retain savings to reinvest in the practice. The significance of turning GPs into fund-holders is that such practices control their own budget, tend to 'shop around' between health authorities in the secondary patient internal market, and are able to reinvest 'profits'. Given such benefits, GP fund-holding will predominate in the primary sector by the year 2000. The doctors' break with the Family Practitioner Committees (later Family Health Service Authorities, then incorporated into the Health Authorities) has effectively made general practitioners into 'medical entrepreneurs'.

- District nurses were designated a crucial role in successful community care implementation. But they increasingly find this to be an impossible task, since the role has been taken out of their purview by the GP fund-holders, by the new community trusts and by the development of skill mix strategies (Groves, 1997). The role of the practice nurse, based in general practice as part of the primary health care team, has expanded even more dramatically to meet the contemporary requirements of community care policy and GP contracting (Green and Saltman, 1997).

- Membership and representation of the Regional Health Authorities and District Health Authorities was restructured. Membership was reduced to five executive members, five non-executive members and a non-executive chair, which in effect meant a removal of locally elected councillors and trade union representatives (Holliday, 1996; Allsop, 1994; Hunter, 1994a; Sullivan, 1996). All of the recommended changes were legalised by their incorporation into the NHS and Community Care Act 1990 for implementation from April 1991.

- In addition, part of the declared aim to improve choice and the quality of health care was the notion of consumer choice. The government declared its commitment to choice and quality for users by reducing restrictions on patients' ability to change their GP, by increasing the proportion of GP income derived from capitation fees, by separating responsibility for purchasing and providing hospital services, and by introducing GP budgets for larger practices (Hunter, 1994a). These aims were absorbed into the published Patients' Charters, produced by local units with what Allsop (1994) describes as 'a confusing mixture of citizen's rights and customer service standards', resulting in 'ultimately a diffusion of responsibility' (ibid. p. 191). Citizens are redefined as consumers (Chapter 10).

Ideology, the new managerialism and the NHS

As we have noted, the health reforms prefigured the future operation of the NHS and related community care strategies. But they are also of major ideological importance in marking a radical change in values which set the agenda for a number of adjacent governmental social policies.

Griffiths 1983 was a watershed, lodged 'as much in the philosophy which shaped its recommendations as in the recommendations themselves. It marked a shift from producer to consumer values' (Klein, 1995, p. 152). Certainly the ideas were radical in their single-minded pursuit of efficiency, a wholesale mode of thinking at the heart of Thatcherism, refashioning the Tory precept that professionals ought to be subject to accountability and control as in the practice of modern businesses (Holliday, 1996). A series of discrete initiatives was already underway in the early 1980s, later fully articulated as the new managerialist philosophy which included the 1980 Korner initiative for new information sytems in the NHS; efficiency savings' targets set by the Secretary of State; the launch of an annual review process; the efficiency scrutinies (by a Marks & Spencer senior executive) of aspects of the public sector; the central control of labour resources; the use of performance indicators; the introduction of compulsory competitive tendering (CCT) for tendering ancillary services; and the compulsory disposal of surplus property – requisite pieces of the considerable NHS estate (Holliday, 1996). In total, these initiatives created a 'frame of mind' for thinking managerially – it was not simply about 'bringing in' managers, although the Griffiths Report was keen on importing the old-style general manager, the conventional private sector business decision maker.

Walby and Greenwell (1994) classify a number of perspectives attached to the new wave management in the NHS through the 1980s. In the first place, the introduction of the general manager reflected the increased influence of Taylorist management. Second was the encouragement of managerial behaviour by senior medical profesionals, effected by greater engagement with the financial mechanisms of medical care – in other words, the increased managerialisation of medicine. Third was the development of a 'new nursing' imbued with holistic modes of treatment and more flexible ways of working, a very different approach from the standardised Taylorist model of management. Fourth, CCT was an attempt to cut costs and control NHS ancillary workers; as such it was resisted vigorously by the unionised workforce, albeit without much success. Fifth was the marketisation of the NHS. Finally, there was the repositioning of the consumer at the forefront by a new wave management attempting to sensitise workers more fully to the consumers' needs, bringing decision making closer to the consumer for greater empowerment.

Marketisation and quasi-markets

We saw above that marketisation forms a key plank in the 'new management' platform, signalling the introduction of business-type internal markets into the NHS and the distinction of buyers and sellers by separating purchasers from providers. Markets and contracts serve to mediate the purchaser:provider relationship. In view of the absence of automatic funding for services offered (for example, by nurse, GP or consultant, as in the past), the very nature of contracts drawn up by the purchasers and providers is integral to the progress of the NHS – contractualism again becomes a more appropriate and necessary way of 'behaving', just one more feature of the complete redirection of health service administration, and one which has also come to dominate social care (Chapter 4).

However, the NHS care markets do not entirely mirror business markets. Contracts are of three basic kinds. With block contracts, the purchaser gains access to a specific range of services before actual delivery. Cost and volume contracts entail a given number of courses of treatment, whereas cost per case contracts operate by the parties involved setting a series of charges for each individual case. While it is the last that most closely resembles the business model, the first type fits into a bureaucratic model. Precisely because of such variations, Le Grand (1990) has labelled these as contractual forms: 'quasi-markets' possessing character-istics diverging from conventional markets in crucial ways. Inde-pendent institutions and public organisations are not necessarily geared towards maximising their profits, and they are not invari-ably privately owned. Consumers do not express their purchasing power in money terms, but in terms of receiving specified allocated resources. In most cases the exercise of choice is not granted to the immediate user, but to a delegated third party, for example a health authority, a GP, or a social services department. 'Welfare quasi-markets' are non-profit organisations which compete for public contracts, sometimes competing with profit-orientated organisations. Consumer purchasing power is centralised into one single purchasing agency, or it is allocated to users through vouchers as opposed to cash. Sometimes consumers are represen-ted in the market by agents rather than functioning on their own (Le Grand and Bartlett, 1993). In the new health quasi-markets, the state's role changes from the old 'bureaucratic' organisation into discrete units of producers and providers of services within a competitive framework.

Consumers, management and choice

Although we have made brief reference to consumerism as part of the new wave management, it is still necessary to explore its ideological meaning. The idea of 'citizens as consumers' became part of the 1991 Citizens Charter launched by John Major, the Conservative Prime Minister, for the improvement of standards in the public sector (Hunter, 1994b). But it was already a feature of the Griffiths health reforms and the 1989 White Paper, and indeed an integral component of the new managerialism. The Conservatives' consumerism manifested the notion of providing individual public service users with greater information, and offering more 'choice' so that the consumer is able to 'exit' from a service and find other alternatives, particularly in the private sector. Clearly, this is not a recipe for consumer participation in management decisions; nor did the consumerist charter represent an extension of legal rights for users of the NHS (Harrison *et al.*, 1992). Rather, it conformed to the market definition of consumer rights.

On the other hand, Community Health Councils have been involved and consumers have been given a voice on Regional or District Health Authorities in areas such as Oxford and South West Thames. Such involvement has nevertheless been at management's behest and has either been ignored or moulded into the 'managerially-malleable form of the survey questionnaire'. 'Notions of direct consumer representation (and still more participation) have no real place in the new provider market' (ibid. p. 138).

Where consumerism, then, is linked with markets and enhanced accountability, evidence points to less accountability with the development of quasi-markets. It has been argued that with the concentration of power in health authorities, scrutiny and accountability of members and managers have declined (Mohan, 1995). 'The opening up of the NHS to market forces,' suggests Mohan, 'and its various administrative reorganisations, has meant that decisions are taken by very few people and without proper scrutiny' (ibid. p. 227).

Apart from the fact that equity and choice have not increased at all in the new NHS, reforms in the direction of new managerialism, flexibility and marketisation have produced operational problems. Administrative costs have grown, yet crucial data for the creation of contracts are not available. Although the government policy of the 1980s spoke much about decentralisation and local autonomy, the central state has dictated the agenda in the 1990s (Allsop, 1994). Health care remains finance driven, but commissioning rules are tight. The number of cases of health authority mismanagement has grown in the new competitive climate. One example was Wessex RHA's failure to control computerisation costs (Allsop, 1994). The health care changes have been largely structural; long-term objectives lag behind. Planning and collaboration, as we shall see are vital to the functioning of any workable community care policy.

To summarise the ideological importance of NHS changes, the underlying move to a managerialist philosophy meant the increased use of business sector techniques in medical care and nursing, a management 'mindset' reinforced by the operation of quasi-markets, contracts and competition in health care, with the state minimised and shorn of its dual purchaser and provider role. The distinct governmental proclamations on consumer citizenship were more about choice than about participation in management decision making or increased accountability in the NHS.

Funding health care

The funding of health care is a basic ingredient in government's drive towards efficiency and the reduction of costs. But in the light of New Right thinking on the necessary reduction of state power, the sources of funding are as relevant as the levels of spending.

The traditional NHS funding is still out of general taxes, and thus partly accountable to Parliament. Indeed only 4 per cent of NHS finances originates from fees and charging (Holliday, 1996). The Review in the 1980s did not attempt to modify this emphasis, a not insignificant action; health has been so intrinsic to the welfare paradigm for the British public that the NHS is perhaps the one area of social policy where the Conservative Government shied away from unequivocal revolutionary privatisation (Sullivan, 1994). A prime tenet of the NHS funding is equal access to health care services according to need rather than ability to pay (Harrison et al., 1990). What is now in dispute is the extent to which the health care reforms of the 1980s and 1990s have in fact displaced this overarching social goal, with their emphasis on cost containment and competitiveness. The principle has been eroded already during the postwar decades – but what of the contemporary picture? (ibid.)

The issue of underfunding

Many of the health reforms changed the direction of funding, through the creation of internal markets and the compulsion for trusts to generate income of their own. Yet whereas the New Right lavished its attentions on the over-liberality of the welfare state's spending on health, the converse is a predominant anxiety over the lack of health funds since the inception of the NHS. Although the total health expenditure has increased rapidly, the UK's total health spending ranked among the lowest in the developed capitalist world at the beginning of the decade (Allsop, 1994; Hill, 1996). A British Social Attitudes Opinion survey (Taylor-Gooby, 1995) testifies to the widespread belief that health care is underfunded by the state. Two crucial factors, however, suggest that this may be an insoluble issue. First is the growing number of users, due to pro-longed average life expectancies, as already noted. Second is the constantly expanding set of expectations of the health service as new technologies are developed, resulting in increased demands placed upon it (Harrison *et al.*, 1990). Health analysts, in assessing the Health 2000 project, have argued that no government is able to fund the NHS sufficiently to meet every demand (Ham and Hewitt, 1995), although we might suggest that there is still much room for improvement.

The growth of private insurance and medicine

The growth of private insurance for health paralleled the increase in the number of private practices during the 1980s. 'For-profit' companies were added to the government backed providence companies such as BUPA at the end of the decade, while the market intensified for private health schemes. Private facilities expanded substantially (Johnson, 1990; Sullivan, 1996), reflecting the increased commercialisation of the hospitals, although still representing less than 10 per cent of national health care. Com-mercialisation grew rapidly after the inception of the 1979 Con-servative Government. Much of this was through the operation of multinational corporations searching for ailing health care systems abroad, but vigorously promoted by the British government (Mohan, 1995). Government tax inducements further encouraged the turn towards the private sector in the 1990s, but were then discontinued under the new Labour Government.

Another shift in methods of funding has produced a major impact upon various communities, affecting the incidence of access to health care, exacerbating other forms of spatial and class disparities. One of the prime changes in the 1989 White Paper was the abolition of the earlier RAWP (Resources Allocation Working Party) formula which was needs-based for allocating health resources based on democratic needs. The new reforms based on the cost-orientated mechanisms of the internal market (which tend to be spatially selective) meant that the more affluent areas of the South East benefited as poorer inner-city areas lost out. Such an 'Adam Smith' type operation of the market's 'invisible hand' is viewed as a politically functional strategy by Mohan (1995) who argues that the reforms were inseparable from the political geography of Conservative government policies since 1979: 'the need to protect core support in the South East appears central to the complaints voiced about subregional resource allocation and to the subsequent proposals' (ibid. p. 100). Later formulae, however, tended to favour London and the disadvantaged regions.

Continuing disparities in access to GPs also compounded these regional inequalities. A 1996 study revealed the Anglia and Oxford health regions with 9.4 per cent more GPs than average, the South and West regions with 7.3 per cent more, and regions such as the North West with 9.4 per cent fewer. A pointed inequality exists in the spatial distribution of practice nurses for primary health care (Hacking, 1996, cited in Brindle, 1996b). Considerable GP disparities also operated in terms of the unequal spread of GP fund-holding adopted by the better organised practices in more affluent areas (Allsop, 1994).

Efficiency, costs and competition

Managed competition itself has exerted a bearing on the area of costs and efficiency (Le Grand and Bartlett, 1993). Studies of GP fund-holding offer mixed evidence as to whether costs are any different under the new system. Benefits of a quasi-market in health and social care, Allsop (1994) argues, tend to be asserted rather than demonstrated. While Enthoven stimulated policy debate, 'analysis of the effect of his ideas on resource allocation and cost control remains incomplete . . . the effects of managed care remain unproven' (ibid. p. 186). Furthermore 'the health service internal market is costly and wasteful', suggests Brindle (1996a).

The goal, then, of funding health through taxation in Britain was challenged by the wide span of the health reforms. But another major task for health services has been the engagement in collaborative care.

Health care, collaboration and community care

A highly pertinent question posed for any analysis of community care is why levels of collaboration have been traditionally so low. Explanation rests partially in the difference of organisational structures between health authorities and social services departments. But it also lies in the realms of ideology: for example, conflicting perspective between health visitors and social workers, or the clash of belief systems and attitudes between GPs and social workers and between hospital consultants and social workers. A study of 236 people in Scotland demonstrates that sets of beliefs and attitudes are supplemented by the incipient organisational *culture*. It concludes that 'the very multiplicity of factors militating against the success of inter-professional working has consequences for attempts to improve collaboration' (Dalley, 1993).

Financial pressures and their very complexities have exacerbated the difficulties of collaboration, causing health and local authorities to adopt defensive postures in defining their discrete responsibilities extremely narrowly (Wistow, 1994, 1995). Thus, the problems of delineating health care from social care have continued (Means and Smith, 1994; Meredith, 1995; Lewis and Glennerster, 1996).

The new community care and collaboration

'Caring For People' and the NHS and Community Care Act demand close collaboration by health agencies with social care and other agencies, because of the pliant boundaries between health and social care. Distinct roles and responsibilities of the health authorities were identified by both the White Paper and the Act. In turn, responsibilities were diverted to the users of services (Means and Smith, 1994; Lewis and Glennerster, 1996).

Implementation of the legislative changes has meant grappling with the major challenges of hospital discharge arrangements, not least the matter of bed blockages in the acute hospital sector which, far from leading to full collaboration, have resulted in conflicts. The 1990 Act indicates the obligation to collaborate. But there is no intrinsic linkage of community care plans with resources allocation, as recommended by the 1988 Griffiths proposals for community care (see Chapter 4 for a fuller discussion). Under Department of Health guidelines, the plans had to be 'based on shared principles and were expected to show how the authorities were going to promote the aims of the legislation in respect of assessing need, clarifying the responsibilities of the agencies involved, securing better value for money, ensuring support for carers and promoting a flourishing independent sector' (cited in Lewis and Glennerster, 1996).

Interdisciplinary assessment of need in community care

'Caring For People' emphasises that assessing individual need, designing care arrangements and securing their delivery are collaborative activities to be carried out with medical, nursing and other agencies. The assessment of need is a complex affair and requires proper interagency collaboration. Bland (1994b) observes that in spite of the policy directives, better interdisciplinary assessment still has some way to go, and suggests that improved interdisciplinary cooperation in assessment calls for an agreed operating framework clarifying such factors as regards:

● the purpose and desired outcomes of interdisciplinary assessments;
● which elements of assessed need are for social or health care;
● which elements of assessment will be handled by which agencies;
● the qualifications and experience of staff involved in interdisciplinary assessment; and
● how to conduct separate assessments where users' and carers' needs conflict.

One of the main failures of the collaborative venture (and community care) was the lack of a direct 'financial imperative' for local authorities to develop joint plans with the NHS (Wistow and Hardy, 1994). This has implied an absence of firm control. A considerable increase in the number of agencies to be coordinated has multiplied problems; authorities within the new purchaser:provider framework have lacked basic 'know-how' for planning such as needs analysis, specification of objectives, setting of standards, and outcome evaluation. Evidently, the potential for successful collaboration and needs-led planning cannot be realised without information collated and fed into the planning process. A host of problems remains, even though the 1980s' joint planning machinery has been modified during the 1990s, in response to the purchaser:provider dichotomy, and retitled 'joint commissioning'.

In the Lewis and Glennerster (1996) study, the erection of formal frameworks for purchasing was crucial, and caused many problems for the authorities, so that informal channels were determining decisions while conflicts between the agencies continued: an unsurprising outcome, since they are 'financed separately, administered separately, staffed by different professions and run within different statutory frameworks' (ibid. pp. 185–6). Indeed, few health and local authorites have held joint ownership over statutory community care plans.

Quasi-markets founded on competition have placed a high premium on collaboration, and hindered the nurturing of trust. The difference in the nature of purchasing structures between health authorities and social services produces difficulties in standardising the formal representation in the joint commissioning structures and in making related decisions. The aims of the two types of authority seem to be at odds with each other under the new system, so that where health authorities are under pressure to remove patients out of beds as quickly as possible, social services' imperatives are to carefully provide assessment and care management (Chapter 4), thus hampering speed of response (Lewis and Glennerster, 1996).

Collaboration, GP fund-holders and GP commissioning

The importance of involving GPs in community care is underlined in various government publications (DoH, *A Framework for*

Community Care Charters in England, 1994; DoH, *NHS Responsibilities for Meeting Continuing Health Care Needs*, 1995, HSG (95) 8, LAC (95) 5; KPMG Peat Marwick, *Delivering the NHS Community Care Agenda*, 1994). However, the GP's role in community care has proved problematic (Elkind *et al.*, 1995).

Hudson (1995) identifes a whole range of tensions experienced by GPs in relation to social work, including the work overload arising from the 1990 legislation, the disparity between the GPs' perceived advocacy role and the inherent rationing entailed in care management, and the effects of discharge of patients from long-stay institutions on the GPs. Such confrontations have highlighted the cultural conflict between social work and general practice. Despite these barriers, collaborative projects such as one in Salford linked single-handed and fund-holding practices with social services via a series of ongoing agreements (Elkind *et al.*, 1995).

If the NHS and social services are to respond flexibly to local health needs and to wield influence over outcomes, argue Shapiro and colleagues (1996), a variety of approaches is needed for involving GPs in commissioning. Investigations in Northumberland, Nottingham, Bromley, Eastern, Wiltshire and Dorset pinpointed good practice in commissioning. The Audit Commission's *What the Doctor Ordered: A study of GP fundholders in England and Wales* (1996) implies that substantial service changes have happened in only a tiny minority of fund-holding practices (Audit Commission, 1996; Chadda, 1996), but Shapiro and colleagues propose that radical cultural shifts have already taken place, especially among the fund-holding GPs who will require support with some of the care provision as the general practice role of care management strengthens, constituting the focal point for primary care in the community (Shapiro *et al.*, 1996).

To summarise, collaboration with social care has been discouraged traditionally by ideological differences in organisational cultures and by financial intricacies. Hence, community care legislation's prioritisation within the health service has caused marked tensions, although the requirements to plan have induced clearer objectives. Close interagency collaboration also constitutes a prerequisite for the new and intricate interdisciplinary modes of assessment. But problems remain for effective collaboration over the reforms, not least in the lack of *formal* planning mechanisms and the absence of joint ownership, the hindrance of quasi-markets and the particular rationale of health services. The collision of cultures also manifests itself in the tensions experienced by GP fund-holders representing the new epicentre of primary health care and in the relationships with social work, but, on the other hand, the number of successful collaborative ventures has grown.

Mental health, illness and attitudes: from institution to community

Mental health is both a central concern for community care policy, and also suggests an archetypal case of the continued dominance of medical autonomy and the medical model adopted by the health services, where practically so many other sets of skills are required. In this sense, we confront the ideological significance of health policies. But in another sense, this policy arena simultaneously reflects and affects social attitudes towards particular health conditions and social groups.

The nature of mental disorder

Within western medicine, the main categories of mental disorder are organic conditions, with physical causes for symptoms such as brain damage, and functional conditions or disorders – neuroses, which are reactions to stress (for example, anxiety, phobias) and psychotic disorders such as depressions and schizophrenia (a brain disorder producing delusions and hallucinations or voices); much of this may be due to inheritance. The condition of dementia, often Alzheimer's disease (a disease of the brain leading to inevitable deterioration of the person) is becoming increasingly germane to service provision, in that it tends to attack people of advanced years. Proportions of very old people have increased substantially in many societies; dementia sufferers, more so than any other people with mental disorders, require growing practical assistance. Indeed, mental disorder is the major reason for people moving into institutional care in old age. Hence, population ageing has dramatically affected mental health services (Murphy, 1991). We may also note that women subject to higher incidences of depression are much more likely to require mental health services (Brown and Harris, 1978; Goodwin, 1990).

The dominance of the medical model in diagnosing illness and treatment in the arena of mental health care is tied to the continued exertion of power by the psychiatry profession and the marginalising of social explanations for mental disorder. Mental distress needs to be understood as a historically and socially constructed disorder, especially for conditions other than the evidently physical/organic diseases such as Alzheimer's. For example, many females facing the huge disparity between their needs and the environment – often 'home' in which they are trapped – experience mental distress (Goodwin, 1990). The ideology of mental health produces far-reaching practical effects. Psychiatrists, party to the social construction, 'have made the diagnosis and ordered the treatment and maintained their power whilst the sufferers such as the alienated housewife who experiences a state of powerlessness and emotional suppression, are administered a course of tranquillisers'. Goodwin concludes: 'the role of the psychiatric profession as an agency of social control becomes clear; its remit is to negotiate and manage the "social construction of reality" of people who "fail" to successfully perform roles required within society' (ibid. p. 41). Such ideological manifestations of psychiatry's medical power bear closely upon the policies relating to institutional and non-institutional care, as well as upon the treatment of minority ethnic groups (Chapter 9).

Institutionalisation or deinstitutionalisation

The recent history of community care, including mental health care policies, mirrors the deinstitutionalisation and demedicalisation of mental health care and the subsequent rundown of the traditional large mental hospital asylums. Major attacks on the institutions from academic quarters emerged in the 1950s and 1960s with extensive policy impacts. Canadian sociologist Erving Goffman's *Asylums* (1961) stands as a seminal work which uncompromisingly characterises the social institution such as the mental hospital as a mode of social control, structured by hierarchy and governed by psychiatrists. This conceptualisation of social control was supported by Foucault's analysis of the asylum's origins (Foucault, 1961, 1973). For Foucault, the birth of the asylums in the nineteenth century represented human beings' mental enchainment: a break with the more humane tradition of the sixteenth and seventeenth centuries.

The alleged oppression of institutionalised medicine and psychiatric power was also assailed by the ideas of anti-psychiatrists such as Laing (1959) in Britain and Szasz (1961) in the United States, drawing attention to the role of others, for instance members of the family, in creating mental distress, and to the role of psychiatrists in upholding the pillars of institutionalised authority. However, their philosophical individualism bordering on eccentricity proved counterproductive, and their influence waned considerably.

A later influence in the intellectual assault on the institutionalisation of mental health was the school of thought arguing for the 'normalisation' of disabilities, based on the ideas of Wolfensburger (1972) and initially developed in relation to service provision for people with learning disabilities. Wolfensburger's revised notion of social role valorisation (SRV) prioritised the value of integration over separation, and used SRV as a tool to change the organisation of services so as to relate to users and their community.

While the idea appears praiseworthy and even uncontentious in the context of community care strategies, it is deeply ideological in its assumption that the social values of the so-called normal community or social group are neutral or uncontestable. After all, what is normal?, 'who is normal?' and are the values and behaviour of the accepted 'normal' society to be aspired to uncritically. These concerns echo those expressed earlier by members of the Laingian anti-psychiatry school (Ryan and Thomas, 1987; Carpenter, 1994).

Deinstitutionalisation

Ironically, the deinstitutionalisation policy, despite its implicit rejection of psychiatry, was accepted early on by the psychiatrists, who were keen to distance themselves from the hospitals. The rundown of the mental hospitals was swift in the 1980s, as we saw in Chapter 2. But the fresh anxiety was that the rundown of long-stay hospitals was being implemented without sufficient provision of care services in the community (Allsop, 1994). No explicit measures were afoot to ensure that patients were not discharged without proper community care, a problem that the Audit Commission (1986) Report, *Making a Reality of Community Care*, deemed particularly acute for mental distress. The mechanisms for redirecting financial resources from health to social care were undeniably faulty, a theme that has consistently beleaguered health–social care collaboration (Chapter 4), and stimulated a Conservative Government Green Paper on 'Mental Health' in 1996.

Lack of replacement of resources in the community following the closure of mental hospitals led to criticisms that the predominant reason for closure was cost saving rather than a restructuring for more humane treatment, a critique reinforced by the legislation of the 1990s. Carpenter (1994) suggests that in the 1990s we might well be witnessing the final realisation of a decarceration process (Scull, 1977) – the early community care on the cheap, where the discharged were simply pushed to the margins of society, resulting in homelessness and often imprisonment. Evidence has accumulated that the disadvantages of a rapid deinstitutionalisation from hospitals have been cataclysmic, problems scarcely diminished by 'Caring For People'. A study of discharged people (Chapman *et al.*, 1991) unearthed no apparent revulsion against treatment in the mental hospitals. Another study of young adults with major psychiatric disorders from the Royal Edinburgh Hospital (Simic, 1994) discovered that patients felt their lives had improved following their exit from the old decrepit Victorian institution. Yet the findings are equivocal. Most remained out in the community and experienced better conditions or simply stable conditions; but others displayed 'severe' mental state or behavioural problems 'resulting in major disruption to their lives, especially towards the end of the follow-up period' (Simic, p. 73).

The more independent model of support produces both organisational and financial difficulties. Provision of mental health services is still riddled with incidents of fruitless collaboration (Means and Smith, 1994). Resettlement of patients discharged from the long-stay mental hospitals remains problematic. Renshaw (1994, p. 84) notes that some 40 per cent of homeless people apparently suffer from major mental distress (more fully discussed in Chapter 7).

A survey conducted in 1990 showed that medical power relocates itself in the community from the hospitals, and that psychiatry continues to hold on to its traditional methods from the base of the smaller district general hospital; drugs and ECT remain 'the dominant responses to emotional distress' (Pilgrim, 1993, p. 250).

Finally, however, such has been the resultant chaos from the community care of discharged mentally ill patients that the Labour Government in 1998 announced its intended reversal of the policy through a proposed Mental Incapacity Bill (*Daily Telegraph*, 17 January 1998).

Organisation of mental health services and the new legislation

In the light of radical reforms, what is the current organisational framework for the provision of mental health services in this country? Apart from the seminal Mental Health Act 1983, national mental health policy remains based on the 1975 White Paper 'Better Services for the Mentally Ill' and its 1985 update. Hence, very little has changed as a result of the 1990 community care legislation. Mental health care is carried out through community mental health centres (CMHCs), asylums, informal carers, voluntary agencies and care management. Community mental health centres developed during the 1980s, and are aimed more at short-term users, who are more articulate, better organised and usually accommodated in converted houses or community-based clinics (Murphy, 1991; Renshaw, 1994). More recently, the centres have devoted greater attention to people with long-term needs, and have become the focus for mental health service provision. For people suffering from acute mental disorder which cannot be handled by family or relatives, 24-hour asylum is offered in acute psychiatric wards within district general hospitals. A significant issue for the hospital service is the maintenance of neither too many nor too few such beds, besides the danger that these beds will be utilised as substitute accommodation for people who have nowhere to go.

As with most other activities labelled community care, relatives act as the main carers in a largely unpaid capacity; and as we discuss elsewhere (Chapter 8), much of this care is carried out by women in highly stressful situations, and frequently lacking 'know-how' or without adequate financial support. Yet Britain's mental health service has for long boasted a well-organised voluntary sector, particularly the National Association for Mental Health (MIND) and the National Schizophrenic Fellowship (NSF). With the 1990 legislation, the active role of such bodies in delivering services directly has substantially increased, but so has the conflict of interests, raising doubts as to the appropriateness of training and the extent to which voluntary agencies should substitute themselves for professional health services.

Although care management, adapted from the initial American case management, is a recent innovation of the social care sector (Chapter 4), more care managers are considered prime facilitators of collaboration and may come from the health sector. Care programmes were formally instituted under the 1990 community care legislation, and involve both the health authorities and local authorities. Therefore, while the general belief is that the social worker is best fitted for the role, others, including health professionals and non-health professionals, may be trained to do the job. Ability to command authority and respect from the pertinent services, such as consultant psychiatrists and housing directors, is what counts in the final analysis (Murphy, 1991).

From 1991 the government allocated a Mental Illness Specific Grant (MISG) to each local authority with the agreement of local health authorities, for the purpose of social care for adults with serious mental health problems (Meredith, 1995). This grant is used for a variety of schemes such as community development and housing projects as well as daily care, domiciliary services and self-help (see Renshaw, 1994, for experiences in Scotland).

Organisational changes in mental health services have generated far-reaching consequences. Hospital rundowns and a more intensive community focus have raised queries respecting the legitimacy of some health care professionals' work, and the need for proper staff development. Central government has been retrogressive in training and retraining arrangements for hospital-based staff employed in the mental health and learning disability fields, which have received low priority locally. Few local authorities possess sufficient expertise for properly supporting people with mental distress in the community, causing further problems of collaboration between health and social care agencies (Means and Smith, 1994). Nor have local authorities displayed great ethnic sensitivity.

Mental health services and racism

Mental health services have proven to be culpable of racism and racial discrimination, stemming from deeply ideological roots, reinforced by a culturally based methodology adopted by mental health practitioners (usually in psychiatry). Such institutional racism is detrimental to people of African-Caribbean and Asian backgrounds. British studies into diagnosis of mental illness (Rack, 1982; Sashidharan, 1989; Knowles, 1991; Fernando, 1991) identify acute disparities in treatment between these minority ethnic groups and the white population, believed to reflect the white, western cultural (and implicitly racist) assumptions underpinning the reigning organic or medical model of mental health (Cowen, 1994). Such assumptions have resulted in disproportionate levels of schizophrenic diagnosis and compulsory detention in mental hospitals under the Mental Health Act 1983 (Littlewood and Lipsedge, 1989; Cope, 1989).

People from minority ethnic groups are more likely to receive inferior mental health provision (Skellington, 1996). As a result of the current community legislation, a high proportion of black people are failing to access mental health services through the 'voluntary admission' channels, which involve referral by GPs to the psychiatrist or to the mental health team. To quote Watters (1996): 'Evidence that Asian people may have difficulty in accessing appropriate services at a primary health care level and "communication difficulties" with GPs indicates that community-based services may be both inappropriate and inaccessible' (ibid. pp. 107–8).

Another aspect of the 1990 Act, which allows the health authorities the jurisdiction as 'purchaser' for deciding on monies allocated for mental health services, marginalises minority ethnic communities still further, as only immediate and major mental health problems are granted assistance. Consequently, less emphasis is placed on making connections with those communities seen as fully utilising services (Watters, 1996).

Comparative health care policies

Many countries' health services have undergone a process of reform in the 1980s and 1990s. Generally, the policies have pursued cost effectiveness as opposed to equity in distribution.

Health care reforms

Health care reforms have taken place in many countries, aimed at ensuring a cheaper and more responsive health care system. A survey of seven European countries (Germany, UK, Belgium,

Netherlands, Spain, France and Ireland) in 1991 revealed a preference for the 'public contract' model of health care, that is, health
care funded globally, but decentralised delivery through the market
(Hurst, 1991, cited in Holliday, 1996).

Holliday (1996) notes that common strategies are being
followed within the global health reform movement, leading to
heightened competition and regulation of institutions and individuals in the care market. New Zealand launched a radical
restructuring of its publicly funded health services in 1991, based
on competitive markets, bidding and contracts, and throwing over
its traditional egalitarian philosophy. But such moves to the political right have been far from unanimous (Ashton, 1995).

The US health care reforms have taken the form of an ongoing
debate. Significantly, President Clinton's ambitious attempt to
adopt a comprehensive health care system was defeated. Hillary
Clinton's 1993 'National Health Care Reform Task Force' had
started from the idea of managed capitalism (propounded by
Enthoven). The aim of managed care was to reduce the costs of
health insurance. Popular pressures led to the Task Force's call for
universal and comprehensive health care, which of course was
resisted by the big business corporations (Navarro, 1994). The
operationalisation of the proposals proved overly complicated
(Beauchamp and Ambrose, 1994; Navarro, 1994). The financial
environment is one of rising medical costs, and more than 24
million people remain totally uninsured for health care. The
evident need in the United States is for a system of national health
insurance (Hackler, 1995). Increasingly, both health insurance and
health care services have been taken over by profit-making companies. But it seems likely that 'by the end of the century a few giant
transnational corporations will dominate the production of health
care in "the new medical-industrial complex"' (Ginsburg, 1992).

Health and social care collaboration

In most West European societies a funding divide stands between
the medical, funded by a national health service or social insurance, and the social, funded by local authorities or social assistance
(Tester, 1996a). Although the social insurance model predomi-
nates in Germany, the sharp divide between social and medical
services means that different types of nursing and home help

receive finance for varying amounts of time, ruled by strict criteria. Problems also exist in coordinating hospital services with home care and ambulatory services, as in Britain. For instance, community care centres may not always be informed that someone needing their services is due for discharge from the hospital (Alber, 1992).

The 1995 Italian health reforms link the public sector more with the private and voluntary sectors. For the past decade, community and home help services have been excluded from national health funding. Yet nursing homes and residential homes' care are subsidised by the country's health service, besides contributions by residents or from social assistance for people on low incomes. But the 1990 local government reforms are expected to exacerbate the health–social services split (Tester, 1996a). In recent years, more attempts have been made to integrate services better through the use of case or care management (on American lines) in France and the Netherlands (Means and Smith, 1994). Even Denmark is now experiencing difficulties in coordinating primary health care and hospitals and social services (ibid.).

With the domination of Medicaid and Medicare funding in the United States, services are highly medically orientated, and thus the health and social services are fragmented. Medicare insurance offers short-term health care for those people with medical needs; also the propensity of the means-tested Medicaid to fund optional community services tends to vary with individual state policy (Tester, 1996a).

Mental health services

The Italian experience of phasing out psychiatric hospitals received acclaim as a strategy for linking health with community care in mental health (Giudice *et al.*, 1991). In response to the post-1980 deinstitutionalisation of psychiatry and the planned establishment of community mental health centres in the regions, the highly successful project in Trieste emphasised the need to change attitudes *within* the hospital, before professional workers and clients move out into the community. Yet the Italian successes were unevenly distributed; community-based services are inadequate in the south, especially those aimed at elderly persons suffering mental distress, and people suffering from depressive illness or long-term psychoses (Means and Smith, 1994).

Comparable health care policy reforms in other economies, then, are posited on welfare mix and decentralised delivery, paralleling the British situation. Ideologically charged by New Right strategies, they also display common problems of health care coordination with local social care organisations and collaborative difficulties between public and private sectors.

Conclusion

In conclusion, we may locate a number of features in the restructuring of health services necessitated by community care reform. First, demographic trends are producing increased demands for long-term health care, largely due to greater longevity; they are also raising questions of health and social care boundaries and respective responsibilities for treatment and care, particularly in the light of challenges to the medical profession's traditional hegemony. Second, the health reforms and legislation represent far more than structural change. At one level Griffiths and the White Paper 'Working For Patients' serve as foundational blocks for the introduction of market mechanisms, internal markets and new cost effectiveness and efficiency measures, and differentiation between purchasers and providers. At a rather deeper level, the reforms are about a way of thinking and behaving, an ideological set of market values which supports the priorities of managerialism and efficiency over the values of welfare, and the philosophy of individualism over collectivism. Third, the funding of health care is clearly a major issue, with the constant spiralling of expectations and the services' inability to meet them through general taxation. The reformulation and privatisation of the funding mechanisms, however, are unlikely to prevent huge inequalities in ability to pay and thus access to health care. Fourth, the statutory duty of health agencies to collaborate in planning and implementing health care in the community is arguably a positive step for clients bewildered by separate sources of provision, but the difficulties experienced in collaborative care signal a resilience of historical professional cultures, especially at the higher tiers of formal decision making. Fifth, the accelerated deinstitutionalisation of mental health care delivery is placing heavier burdens on the independent sector to meet care in the community in the absence of realistic funding.

74

There is a crisis of confidence in professional skills 'out in the community'. At the same time, groups in the community such as African-Caribbeans suffer from insensitive forms of mental health care delivery and new allocation procedures. Finally, the common trajectory of health care reform among western capitalist economies reinforces business behaviour and responsiveness to 'choice' in the restructuring of institutions and the values of welfarism in the public sector. The next chapter will investigate the parallel changes in social care, shaped by the same managerialist philosophy of welfare provision, which prefigured an almost unprecedented overhaul of local authority welfare services.

Further reading

Skidmore, D. (1997) (ed.) *Community Care: Initial training and beyond*, London: Arnold. Separate contributors focusing on issues for health professionals in community care.

Mohan, J. (1995) *A National Health Service? The Restructuring of Health Care in Britain since 1979*, London: Macmillan. Places the reforms in their ideological context.

Leff, J. (ed.) (1997) *Care In The Community: Illusion or reality?*, London: Wiley. Collection covers a wide range of issues relating to mental health care.

Wall, A. (ed.) (1996) *Health Care Systems in Liberal Democracies*, London: Routledge. A useful comparison of evolving patterns of health care in Western European, British, American and Australian economies.

4
SOCIAL SERVICES, COMMUNITY CARE AND THE MARKET

Introduction

Social care services for community care have been touched by the governmental social policy climate in ways directly comparable with the health service changes. The de-emphasis of state provision severely marginalised the traditional *modus operandi* of social services, not least because of continuing cutbacks in real public social expenditure (George, 1996), but also because of the new 'imperatives' in the turn towards the market and 'welfare mix'. The adoption of the New Right philosophies calling for a refocusing upon individual, family and 'community' meant a reduced autonomy for local authority social services departments now transformed into enabling agencies relating to other independent and quasi-state providers (Sullivan, 1996).

It has been argued that the broader global shifts entailing new post-Fordist and post-modern organisational forms of production may mean a novel flexibility of service delivery (Loader and Burrows, 1994), but debate turns on whether new cost-conscious market-driven services are appropriate or serve the activity of social care. As we shall see in this chapter, managerialism and market relationships inform virtually all changes in social and community care. The chapter examines the models of community care traditionally operated by social services. It then describes the landmarks of the current community care legislation, and the concomitant restructuring of local authorities and social services. A closer examination discusses the full implications of the purchaser:provider split for social care; the role of the voluntary and independent sectors; the crucial changes in the funding of social care; the significance of community care plans; care management and assessment; the changing conditions of social work; and finally, the international experience.

Models of care

Traditionally, three main types of community care are provided by social services: day care, residential care and domiciliary care. Their significance has changed with the more recent community care legislation. But to bring into focus the full measure of social services' or state involvement in caring, we must also consider the continued importance of the 'informal caring' offered by families, fundamentally carried out by women, and which represents the best part of caring performed in the society.

Day care

Social services departments have run day centres for the client groups requiring community care, and for their families. Day care is intended to support people remaining in their own home. The range of day care services includes adult training centres (ATCs), which have been aimed at people with learning difficulties, gaining educational and workshop experience. While their depressing environments and restricted access to fully paid work have been subject to considerable criticism, new ventures and directions were developed in the late 1980s (for example, sheltered work groups and workers' cooperatives), but work opportunities remain scarce (McNally and Rose, 1994).

Social and recreational day centres exist for persons registered and disabled, offering social contact with the world outside the home and for mentally distressed people. Day care facilities have been available for elderly people at local residential homes, as well as for residents. However, separate community resources and day centres have been developed for a variety of purposes. McNally and Rose (1994) note the increasing need for handling a range of special care. Current facilities are proving inadequate to deal with the closure and contraction of hospitals and the associated growth

77

in numbers of people with profound and multiple disabilities, plus older people with a learning disability who require a day service and are particularly socially isolated.

Residential care

Residential care services cover elderly persons' homes and residential establishments for people with learning difficulties, people suffering from mental distress, and residential homes for severely physically handicapped people unable to look after themselves at home and without alternative caring support. Residential care homes, subject to strict inspection, are registered under the Registered Homes Act 1984, but other types of residential care accommodation include staffed hostels, which vary in their staffing levels, and group homes under schemes for shared living whereby people with mental health difficulties or learning difficulties share a house with non-disabled tenants and receive support from the latter. Residential homes have also been provided by the private and voluntary sectors, although the state still met the costs through the social security benefits system. And it is precisely the topic of funding that proved the catalyst for the community care reforms, powered by the need to 'stop the haemorrhage in the social security budget . . . (like) the Health Service reforms . . . pushed through to meet a crisis ' (Lewis and Glennerster, 1996, p. 8).

The numbers of local authority-owned or -financed residential homes have fallen drastically; social services departments have become the prime purchasers of residential care within a managed market (discussed below) with the new legislation and the changing role of local authorities. New funding arrangements, the more pronounced emphasis on independent living and the shift to independent and private sector provision under the mixed economy have totally altered the profile of residential care (Alaszewski and Wun, 1994). One undisputed consequence is a severe reduction in choice for public sector residential care.

Domiciliary care

Social services departments have provided domiciliary support, aimed at assisting clients and carers living at home. Such services comprise home helps allocated to people in the community who are ill-equipped to carry out certain tasks. This provides much needed social contact for elderly people, while also monitoring the client's general demeanour. Significantly, however, the new legislation has produced difficulties in terms of the precise identification of those tasks which require health care input on the one hand and social care on the other – for example, who bathes a client? Nor have substantial improvements in user-orientated care resulted, such as being put to bed at a preferred time (Lewis and Glennerster, 1996).

Domiciliary care services may also include special night-sitting support to physically handicapped and elderly persons living in their own physically adapted homes. However, the government's severe cuts in housing expenditure included reductions in available monies for disabled facilities grants (Meredith, 1995). Ironically, with the increased popularity of such dwellings, spending cuts have led to reductions in the numbers of wardens for elderly and handicapped persons inhabiting sheltered accommodation in independent living units. 'Meals-on-wheels' services are not delivered daily, but represent a supplement to the expected family or informal neighbourly input. Many authorities display a continuing insensitivity towards the specific dietary requirements of people from black and minority ethnic groups, especially respecting the lack of any vegetarian food or halal meat or the poor day care provision (Atkin and Rollings, 1996).

Informal family care

As we have already noted, the greatest part of caring is carried out informally either by family or neighbours, usually the former: women tend to constitute a large proportion of family carers. Indeed, the economy and social welfare services have depended upon this vital yet unpaid task of domestic labour, entailing looking after sick and disabled members of the family (Manthorpe, 1994).

Informal care also brings enormous financial costs for the carer, not least the lost opportunity costs of income from employment. Without compensation from the state, the latter gains by an estimated £15–34 billions annually. Community care policy has tended to perpetuate the exploitation, given the greater emphasis placed on care *by* the community, while intensifying the differentials in incomes and employment opportunities between men and women.

Current community care policy under the Carers' (Recognition and Services) Act formally recognises the needs of carers who previously remained more or less invisible. 'Caring For People's major objectives accorded high priority to practical social providers' support for carers. Carers are accepted as 'important', willing, and 'deserving of help' (Manthorpe, p. 115). They now enter into the assessment and care management procedures analysed later in the chapter. New approaches to carer support are calculated to facilitate greater flexibility, through flexible care attendance schemes, neighbourhood care schemes, home-based flexible respite care, plus information, advice and support. To sum up, all main forms of formal care have experienced marked change; the scale of unpaid informal care, however, remains a crucial cost-saving activity for the state, an outcome no doubt assumed by the legislation itself.

The community care legislation

The British Conservative Government's community care legislation was emblematic of the New Right social policy agenda. Policy statements, papers and Acts throughout the 1980s and 1990s transformed the face of social care provision, while complementing the equally radical reforms of the Health Service firmly underpinned by managerialism, markets and contracts.

Audit Commission and Griffiths 1988

In 1985 the Parliamentary Select Committee on the Social Services announced its disquiet with the general lack of progress in community care policies and the public concern at the high proportion of discharges from mental hospitals lacking follow-up care. The Audit Commission's (1986) cost-effectiveness investigation, *Making A Reality of Community Care*, demonstrated the government's inability to implement community policies nationwide, and focused too easily on the facility of social security for enabling people to enter residential care at government expense (Payne, 1995).

The 1988 review of community care (the second half of a combined health and social care strategy) was conducted by a business

Box 4.1   Government statements and legislation on community care

1986 *Audit Commission*: Making a Reality of Community Care

1988 *Local Government Act*:
– Certain services to be put out to competitive tender.
– Encouraged residential homes in private sector.

1988 *Wagner Report*:
– Called for system of registration and inspection for local authority, voluntary and private residential homes.

1988 *Griffiths Report*: Community Care: Agenda for action
– Recommended switch of financial responsibility for community care to local authorities.
– Stress on informal carers, voluntary groups and private voluntary sector.

1989 *Government White Paper*: *'Caring For People'*
– Proposals built on Griffiths Report.
– Shift of costs to local authorities.
– 'Market relations' within the social services.
– Creation of six 'key responsibilities for social services'.
– Special responsibilities for health authorities.

1990 *NHS and Community Care Act*
– Amended 1948 National Assistance Act.
– Local authority to prepare community care plans.
– Duty to assess people potentially in need of community care services.
– Local authorities' added powers to inspect their residential homes.

1991 *Government (DoH) policy guidance*: Community Care in the Next Decade and Beyond

1992 *Audit Commission*: (a) Community Care: Managing the cascade of change; (b) The Community Revolution: The personal social services

1993 *Formal care management implementation of 1990 NHS and Community Care Act by local authorities*

1995 *Carers' (Recognition and Services) Act*

executive, Sir Roy Griffiths. His final report, *Community Care: Agenda for action*, advocated a mixed economy and the development and regulation of community care. At the heart of the recommendations lay the modernisation of management, an importation of managerialism equivalent to the one he advocated earlier for the Health Service. Griffiths proposed a minister empowered with monitoring national and local policies. The Report's 'welfare mix' approach entailed a widening of service provision to encompass bodies from the private and voluntary sectors, so as to 'widen consumer choice, stimulate innovation, and encourage efficiency' (Griffiths, 1988, para. 1.3.4). Local authority social services were to redefine their role from providers to enablers and facilitators. Other role redefinitions required fundamental changes for certain occupational and professional groups like social workers.

The 1989 White Paper: 'Caring For People'

'Caring For People' constituted the social care equivalent of the government's 'Working For Patients' for the health services (see Chapter 3). It set out six primary objectives: services for people at home; services for carers; assessment for care (through individual packages of care); 'a mixed economy of public and independent sector care', 'to make social services "enabling" agencies'; clear delimitation of agency responsibilities; and better value for taxpayers' money.

The White Paper explicitly articulated the roles and responsibilities of health authorities, reflecting anxiety over the long-standing health and social care split. These authorities were to remain responsible for the health care needs of people who also required social care, while the primary responsibility for the community health services would stay with the District Health Authorities. In addition, the White Paper expected Health Authorities and Family Practitioner Committees to contribute specifically to the new arrangements for community care, including close collaboration with social services for assessment, preparation of community care plans, and presentation of policies for intended community services and care.

GPs were also the subject of expected local agreements enabling them to contribute fully to community care. Community nursing staff, including district nurses, health visitors, and community psychiatric and 'mental handicap' nurses, were to make a substantial contribution to community care development through involvement with care arrangements, assessment procedures and the provision of care in the wake of care package design. Health authorities were invested with initial responsibility to plan for highly dependent persons' long-term care; this has become a contentious area because of the financial implications as to where long-term care is carried out.

Among the key changes signalled by the White Paper was the responsibility of social service authorities for the design of care packages for clients within the available budget – transparent indication of a cost-driven strategy closely controlled under care management. A new specific grant was introduced for promoting the development of social care for seriously ill people, available to local authorities for projects agreed with the local health authorities. 'Caring For People' proposed that local authority social services departments set up new complaints procedures; further, local authorities were instructed to institute a system of inspection and registration for residential homes in all sectors, 'at arms-length from the management of their own services'.

Although the White Paper's proposals basically mirrored the Griffiths recommendations of 1988, unlike Griffiths they did not advocate a Ministry of Community Care or set aside special funds clearly targeted at social care. Instead, the extra financing was to be achieved through transferring monies out of the social security budget and by affording to local authorities discretion over how much of their budget should be spent on community services (Means and Smith, 1994).

The 1990 NHS and Community Care Act

The main changes contained in 'Caring For People', along with 'Working For Patients', were consolidated and made law by the NHS and Community Care Act 1990. In conjunction with the Act, the government issued the policy guidance *Community Care in the Next Decade and Beyond*, setting out how local authorities should effect the 1989 reforms and the 1990 Act. Implementation of the Act was immediately subject to major delays; the mental health grant and the complaints procedures were due for April 1991; community care plans would not be a statutory requirement until

April 1992, whereas the government rescheduled the transference of social security payments for residents to 1993. One might argue that much of the delay was connected not only with the paucity of funding for such a major set of reforms, but also with uncertainties as to the precise delineation of responsibilities. Joint planning guidance, despite governmental intentions, meant that neither health authorities nor local authorities were prepared for complete implementation, even by April 1993, not least in those local authorities whose social services departments were undergoing total restructuring (Means and Smith, 1994; Malin, 1994).

Social services had become the lead agency for community care under the Act, but in close collaboration with the health authorities and holding a brief to match individual needs with available resources. The new framework was a market-orientated model comprising a network of purchasers and providers: a strategy of 'containment' of costs while offering more services (Payne, 1995). As we shall see below, social services' reconstituted duties not only drastically transformed social service organisations, but redefined professional social work almost beyond recognition.

The restructuring of social services and local authorities

Social services, central to community care strategy, had to be fundamentally restructured in the wake of the reforms. Such restructuring, however, must be grasped in relation to broader capitalist economic restructuring processes, the major restructuring of local government in the 1980s and 1990s, and the dominance of managerialism. A wealth of literature is available on the economic restructuring of the capitalist economy in the 1980s (e.g. Harvey, 1989; Cooke, 1989; Massey, 1995). As we discussed in Chapter 1, post-Fordist tendencies and New Right political policies may explain the new landscape of the state sector, affecting the whole system of social policy making, the public sector and welfare provision. Decision-making processes and welfare-related organisations have become decentralised but fragmented (Harloe *et al.*, 1990). The local welfare state has been restructured so as to facilitate or manage economic development and financial effectiveness, as opposed to meeting welfare needs (Cochrane, 1993).

Strategic management has risen to prominence in local government *per se*: new management borrows the language of enterprise from the private business sector. It emphasises interorganisational working and collaboration with the public, private and the voluntary (non-profit) sectors. New management in local government parallels the new role identified for local authorities as 'enabling authorities', and invests senior managers and chief officers with a higher profile under the government legislation.

New managerialism and the restructuring of social services

Local social services departments have been heavily subjected to radical change, marketisation and managerialism, effectively an assault on professional cultures (Clarke, 1996; Clarke and Newman, 1997). For social services, this has produced sharp repercussions for the social work profession's working conditions and trade union rights (discussed in a later section). New social services structures have resited their centre of gravity from professional to managerial control. Agents of change are juxtaposed to professionalism and administrative bureaucracy; a preoccupation with customer and client (concepts culled from the consumerist language of the business world) replaces the inflexibility of the alleged bureaucratic procedures of the old welfare state public sector.

Already in place within the private sector, the new management model, rendered feasible by developments in financial information systems and computerised management, promotes centralised control over values, culture and strategy and the devolution of control over day-to-day management. Such changes in the technology of management facilitated the new structures for social services and their redefined role as 'enablers', linked to the displacement of the public sector's dominance by market relationships and the ideology of the mixed economy (Lawson, 1993).

Markets and social care services

Managerialism is a natural adjunct to the marketisation of social services and welfare. Use of the market model is intended to instil the spirit of competition in social services departments as they transform themselves from universal providers to actors in a business climate of purchasers and providers, as in the health service. The operation of internal markets, where units *within* local authorities compete with one another, is harnessed to this model of organisations competing with external contractors (Clarke, 1996). Yet where one might conclude that public welfare provision has been taken over by markets and private competition, 'quasi-markets' imply that the state has not been replaced. Rather, what remains of state welfare has been reconstructed to mimic the market through the creation of quasi-markets and quasi-customers (Clarke and Langan, 1993). In the light of such global factors, social services departments have had to reorganise, often tentatively and reluctantly, in order to reflect the purchaser:provider splits, care management functions, quality assurance procedures and mixed welfare provision (Hoyes and Means, 1993b; Wistow *et al.*, 1994; Means and Smith, 1994).

Lewis and Glennerster's (1996) detailed examination of the responses of five authorities (metropolitan and county) in the reorganisation of their social services unearthed substantially diverse approaches and speed of implementation. Notwithstanding, each has moved towards the creation of a distinct functional division between purchasing and providing sections. Community care directives, in this respect, have culminated in fundamental restructuring on the ground. They have transformed social services departmental cultures in two basic ways: first, by incorporating the imperative to be 'enablers', not 'doers'; second, by acting on the imperative to institute systems which demand managerial skills. This has completely redirected the work of social services departments, although smaller social work departments as in Scotland are less likely to possess the resources and the expertise to stimulate the market in the independent sector and thus effectively to deliver community services (McGarvey and Midwinter, 1996).

The restructuring of local authorities and social services, then, resembles developments previously specific to private manufacturing; its subsequent application to local government has led to an upgrading of strategic management and the promotion of efficency and cost-effective measures. The managerial model in social services has not only been used to restructure services, but also to substitute care professional values with those of a new style of quasi-market which encourages competitive behaviour and choice rather than 'profit'. On the other hand, widespread opposition in social care to the restructuring expresses not only frustration at a restrictive climate of resource cutbacks, but also the belief that one ought not to treat health and welfare as consumer commodities.

The purchaser:provider split in social services

The newly reorganised activities of purchasing and providing, whereby the providers of a social service are no longer synonymous with the purchasers, must be seen in relation to the redefinition of social service authorities as enabling authorities, operating in a market environment and contracting for services as discussed below. As we have observed, both the community care reforms and those for the health services (see Chapter 3) have changed their role of provider to one of enabler. Essentially, this means that instead of directly providing services such as day or residential care themselves, the authorities are expected to arrange services made available by a range of providers. These may well include the local authority itself, but should also embrace organisations in the private and voluntary sectors, that is, the 'mixed economy of care'. The role of enabler is to offer a greater choice of services than hitherto, to encourage competition between providers, and to stimulate the independent sector to provide community services (Meredith, 1995).

The purchaser:provider split refers to the organisational divisions made by the local authorities to reflect the new emphasis upon purchasing and contracting. Just as the health authorities redirected responsibility for provision of services towards the newly created, separate NHS trusts, some local authorities – for example, Tameside, Somerset and Cheshire – transferred key services such as day care, residential homes and home helps to specially formed organisations such as trusts or various 'not-for-profit' companies (Meredith, 1995).

From the inception of the reforms, social services departments experienced difficulties not so much with the prospect of purchasing services and using outside suppliers – often the case – but with the scale of necessary arrangements such as setting up information systems to speedily effect the purchaser:provider split (Rao, 1991; Wistow *et al.*, 1994). Negotiating the new purchaser:provider relationships has proved difficult for authorities, creating tensions with the breaking down of formerly professional jurisdictions, and the search for a new role in purchasing divisions. The Lewis and Glennerster (1996) survey found that the purchasing function and the adjacent specialised management divisions such as care management and commissioning units were slow in taking shape. Government offered slight policy guidance for developing purchasing strategies. Viable strategies and stimulation of the independent sector necessitate sophisticated access to market information. Performance in practice differed between the authorities, although they all experienced large barriers in the technical tracking of the market without available skills. Increased workload and related stress resulted from the purchaser:provider dichotomy.

Contracts and the social care market

An essential ingredient of the purchasing function is the requirement to set up contracts; 85 per cent of new SSD spending must be in the independent sector. Following the 1993 implementation of the Act, the move from local authority to independent provision was dramatic in home care and residential care (Lewis and Glennerster, 1996). Admittedly there was nothing novel in social services departments dealing with external contractors, but what *is* new is the contractual basis determining all aspects of the relationship, including grants and dispute procedures. This is cause for concern for voluntary agencies whose futures may seem increasingly threatened. Contracting with the private sector has grown substantially, especially in private home care provision (Flynn, 1996; Flynn *et al.*, 1996). In some areas the private sector has established itself as a provider of domiciliary care generally through small businesses offering a 'flexibility' which encompasses long or inconvenient working hours (Meredith, 1995).

Contractual obligations built into the purchaser:provider split were intended to encourage greater choice for service users, and to bring about the extension of consumers' rights. However, consumers' rights with contracted community care services are not safeguarded in the same way as goods directly changing hands for cash, since the contractual relationship is between the purchaser and the provider. And it is precisely this concept of user empowerment that is encouraging the greatest scepticism, considering the marginalisation of many user groups in the purchaser:provider mode of operation (see Part II for a more detailed discussion of user groups and empowerment). Lewis and Glennerster (1996) failed to identify any real increase in choice and responsiveness to client needs resulting from contractual operations in the social care market, but did encounter an intimidating growth of bureaucracy and a maintenance of institutional expenditure.

The role of voluntary and independent sectors

We noted in Chapter 2 the historical significance of the voluntary sector and its key role in the development of welfare services in Britain. But because of the expanding diversity within the sector, it is no longer easy to define or identify voluntary organisations which are neither part of the state nor accountable to local elected state representatives; while they are private bodies, they are not commercial, profit-seeking organisations (Alcock, 1996). Ostensible boundaries of the voluntary, state, market and informal sectors nevertheless overlap, posing a challenge to those voluntary organisations positioned on the periphery.

The Griffiths Report (1988, para. 8.11) outlined the roles of voluntary sector bodies as self-help, information provision, befriending, advocacy, public education, campaigning, innovating and monitoring, in addition to service provision. With the 'contracts' policy for the mixed care economy, many voluntary bodies find themselves on the horns of a dilemma whereby their contracts tie them more securely to the state and inhibit their independent and critical roles (Meredith, 1995). Such tensions endanger the very strength and nature of the partnership envisaged by the government (Reading, 1994; Alcock, 1996).

Restructuring of the welfare state, contracts and the politics of the voluntary sector

The voluntary sector ranges from huge national charities to tiny self-help groups. Services offered vary from day care to counselling to housing and shelter (Reading, 1994; Taylor *et al.*, 1995). Whereas this diversity is no doubt healthy and to be encouraged, a survey by Taylor and colleagues (1995) pointed to growing pressures in the opposite direction: towards growth, formalisation and standard modes of operation, pressures reinforced by the incipient managerialism and the mode of community care implementation.

Governmental moves to the market and the contract culture during the late 1990s in community care have exerted profound political repercussions, not least in restating the relationship between the statutory and voluntary sectors and the formalisation referred to above. Reading (1994) argues that the political teeth of voluntary organisatons have been extracted; their direct responsiveness to the service user is endangered as they become totally reliant on the local authorities for finance (Reading, 1994; Wistow, 1994). Their existence is uncertain and problematic with the change from grants to contracts or service agreements. New business methods of working are now imposed upon voluntary organisations. Fresh management skills are expected of their workers as problems arise in dealing with the new social service department structures and with protracted contract negotiations (Lewis and Glennerster, 1996). But markets do not necessarily complement the traditional responsiveness of local 'MIND' groups (Nicholls, 1997).

The formalisation of grant aid has encouraged greater professionalisation among voluntary bodies; it has influenced their operations and accountability, and prime goals such as targeting highly dependent client groups. If anything, voluntary organisations are having to become more bureaucratic. The higher profile of voluntary organisations affects working conditions for employees in a sector unused to maintaining good working conditions. As more workers become employed in this sector, the intensification of negotiated contracts raises a host of trade union issues (Carpenter, 1994).

Despite early promises in official statements, the sector's robustness is impaired by the cumulative effects of major cuts in social services budgets. Annual financial cutbacks in the order of 8 per cent in real terms have an immediate bearing upon service users. For example, elderly and disabled persons, affected by reductions in direct social services, find that the services they tend to rely on soon disappear as projects are shelved by the new voluntary providers, ironic in that the projects include those aimed at enabling people to remain in their own home under community care policy! (Cervi, 1996).

Community care and black organisations

Community care policy developments and their impact on voluntary organisations affect black communities in specific ways, given the success of black voluntary organisations. As we have seen, the community care legislation recognised the particular needs of minority ethnic groups as of symbolic interest; it arrived at the point of a major services restructuring, just when the gulf widens between 'evident need and available resources' (Walker and Ahmad, 1994, p. 66). Black voluntary organisations are diverse and well established, primarily due to the lack of adequate statutory and voluntary service provision for black communities. The latter have had to provide for their own wide and general set of needs. Development of black voluntary organisations, in particular the black housing movement and the introduction of black housing associations through the 1980s and 1990s, is recognised as a positive achievement within the voluntary sector. In addition, their five-year plans received backing from the Housing Corporation (Reading, 1994; Harrison, M., 1993, 1995, 1996).

In spite of these achievements, market strategies in advancing social care are problematic for the black voluntary groups. Black voluntary provision remains generally underresourced and underdeveloped, in danger of being pushed aside by large national or private voluntary care agencies, because of the paucity of social services support and an absence of enforcement of anti-discriminatory clauses in contract specifications. Intensified spending cutbacks reinforced by institutional racism demonstrate the inherent barriers for black voluntary groups to survive or to cultivate the requisite professionalism for competing in a contract culture which measures success financially. They are in a worse position for competing on equal terms, while community care policy prioritises the longer-established traditional voluntary groups (Walker and Ahmad, 1994; Atkin, 1996).

But such a prognosis seems unduly pessimistic for some analysts. With the vagaries of the mixed care market, it is crucial that minority ethnic groups and black organisations are able to take advantage of the possible opportunities for empowerment, and ensure prioritisation through continued struggle for equal rights and treatment (Reading, 1994; Atkin, 1996). Nevertheless, as a recent Commission report argues, the lack of access to funds remains an urgent matter for the future. Loraine Martins, director of the black groups' umbrella organisation, declares that, 'Black people are not even at the starting block, because they are not getting the funding' (Francis, 1996c, p. 19; Whiteley and Valios, 1996).

Although Griffiths defined their specific roles, voluntary organisations are bound to the state more than ever through a contracting process which compromises their previous independence, standardises and bureaucratises their operations, reduces their political influence, yet enhances their professionalism. Withdrawal of social services resourcing means the annulment of voluntary projects aimed at community care user groups, and the demise of once buoyant black voluntary organisations. Finally, although the potential exists for greater empowerment and equal rights under the legislation, the record so far suggests a more cautious note.

The funding of social care

Funding social care is, of course, a central issue in governmental community care policy, not least because of the demographic projections of older people requiring care, and government's anxiety to control the growth in public expenditure. The restructuring of health and social services and the shifting of responsibilities from central government bodies to local authorities entails the reorganisation of financial arrangements for caring for people at home, community health care and the independent sector.

New funding mechanisms for community care

The community care reforms involved major cash transfers from national level (DSS) to local authorities, and special arrangements for people on income support. Negotiation of the exact amounts for transfer to and distribution among local authorities was certainly complicated, with prior spending on residential and nursing home care of more than £2.5 billion through the government income support system. However, a crucial factor in the transfer was that the financial support transfer system was for three years only. Since 1997, local authorities have had to rely upon other sources (Meredith, 1995; Lewis and Glennerster, 1996).

The sums transferred to local authorities for the early years following the formal implementation of the 1990 Act are the product of calculations of how much the central government would have spent on care in homes in the past, less the sum the Department of Social Security will still need to spend on people in homes (including a new residential allowance and ordinary Income Support). Taking into account other sums – for example, administration of the Independent Living Fund – a Special Transitional Grant (STG) of some £518 million was provided by 1996 to local authority social services, for spending on the new specific community care responsibilities. A further condition, reflecting the 'mixed economy of care' philosophy, was that 85 per cent of the grant's social security element had to be spent with the independent sector. (Other specific grants included one for mental health.)

Payment arrangements for care for people in their own home

What of paying for care in people's own homes, as opposed to care in care homes? After 1993, the old system of charging for 'non-residential social services' (or day and domiciliary services) remained roughly the same as before. Every local authority was empowered to set its own charges at a 'reasonable' level; where the person has insufficient means to pay for themselves, the local authority may demand what is considered 'practically feasible' following a needs and financial assessment. Government expected the local authority to raise 9 per cent of its non-residential social services through charges. This creates the dilemma of either charging prohibitive rates and thus dissuading people from seeking help to stay in their own home (a priority aim of the community care policy) or raising insufficient funds to facilitate sufficient care. Wide disparities appear in authorities' charging policies. Government policy is for local authorities not to exempt people on income support from charges.

An added anomaly exists within the charging policy. With the pressures mounting for local authorities to raise more of their own income and continued restrictions on budgets, local authorities impose high charges for their non-residential services. Furthermore, the disparity between residential and non-residential charging systems is leading authorities to place people in care homes rather than provide home care. The value of a person's own property is only taken into account for care homes, which seems to run counter to the supposition that care in the community is a cheaper option (Meredith, 1995).

The basis for charging has been unclear, yet authorities now charge for a wider range of services at higher prices. A study of six local authorities found charging policies to be unfair and based on unreasonable assumptions, for instance that clients in fact received basic living allowances through income support, or that clients were able to use attendance allowance towards part of the cost of their services, or that savings were solely available to pay for services (Baldwin and Lunt, 1996a, 1996b). Many of the steeper charging policies were in response to increasing financial pressures with the rising demands for services and health authorities 'cost-shunting' their piece of the funding by redefining community services as 'social' care.

The increasing numbers of people requiring community health services in the home due to ageing and justified by the new community care policy have created a new client group whose responsibility is evidently neither that of health nor of social care services. Such ambivalence in turn poses the question of which service should bear the cost – a prime aspect of the health–social care collaborative arrangements and the ability to monitor developments (Means and Smith, 1994; Meredith, 1995).

The crisis in community care funding and levels of resources

One heavy irony of the community care policy is that its inauguration at the start of the decade with the burgeoning demand for care was followed by the precipitate declaration of crises in community care funding and restrictions upon local financial autonomy. Accusations were made that the policy was a cynical exercise to negate the allegedly progressive features of delivering care. Chances of adequate funding for local authorities were slender (Hudson, 1995). Many authorities came under severe pressure by the mid-1990s because of the cut in the government's revenue support grant (Lewis and Glennerster, 1996; George, 1996).

A widely publicised case in point was the 1996 Appeal Court judgment against Gloucestershire County Council's community care cutbacks in resources. Local authorities were instructed not to

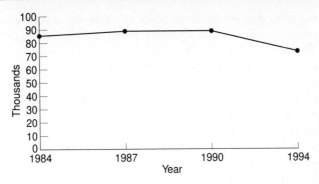

Figure 4.1 Numbers of residential care staff in England 1984–1994. (Source: *Social Trends*, 1996.)

use lack of resources as justification for a reduction in services (Cooper, 1996). Owing to the budgetary restrictions the ruling meant that thousands of disabled persons whose services were withdrawn or cut back were now entitled to their restoration. However, the decison was yet again reversed by the House of Lords judgment in 1997, much to chagrin of the disability rights movement (*Guardian*, 21 March 1997).

Community care policy, then, has instituted new mechanisms for its funding. Whereas substantial cash transfers supported localities in the first instance, the full burden now falls on local authorities, and especially on those with poorer populations. Higher charging ironically leads to downgrading of support for home care; at the same time, clients have become a football between health and social care agencies. Local authorities' distinct inability to meet the users' requirements during the late 1990s gives the lie to claims of enhanced client empowerment.

Community care plans

Production of community care plans represents a key procedural task legally imposed upon local authorities' social services, an exercise covering a number of providing agencies. Local authorities have to prepare, publish and monitor a community care plan (under Section 46 of the 1990 Act) in concert with other agencies, and to include identification of the total population's needs, existing services and plans for people at home, methods of increasing consumer choice and stimulating the operation of the mixed economy of care and consultation. They must also incorporate the requisite costings and staffing and publicising of their plans, indications of resourcing and increasing the involvement of service users and carers, developing assessment and care management systems, extending joint working between health and social services, involving other agencies, shifting the balance of resources towards non-residential care, and providing more respite care and support for carers (Meredith, 1995).

Linking and collaboration in community care plans

The engagement of social services with other agencies was an essential feature of the local plans. Thus linkages with the District Health Authority, the Family Health Services Authority, the housing authorities and also housing associations, voluntary housing agencies and voluntary organisations representing users of services or their carers, as well as private sector providers, were crucial. The proposed collaboration in the plans served as a mode of government control. Wistow and Hardy (1994) suggest that tying resource allocation to the submission of collaboratively formulated plans was 'an attempt to design accountability and control processes which could secure concerted action at the local level consistent with national policy objectives and priorities' (ibid. p. 48). Collaboration, however, has remained patchy and problematic (Chapter 3 and Lewis and Glennerster, 1996).

Another key aspect of community care planning is the aim for consultation with users, carers and local organisations including representatives of independent providers. The consultation process was expected to demonstrate active responses to the views of users and also potential users. But again the results have been uneven. It is doubtful whether users have been more involved overall in strategic plan-making, such as in the formal collaborative machinery; the level of success varies between authorities (Lewis and Glennerster, 1996).

Community planning may easily become routinised into the cycle of committee meetings and come to depend on how much the preparation of one community care plan encompasses the complex series of needs. Frequently, local authorities fail to consult with private sector providers out of a reluctance to work alongside them (Meredith, 1995), symptomatic of tensions arising in the 'mixed economy' of care.

In demonstrating responsiveness to the 'consumer', local authorities must collaborate with housing, health and other organisations for the production of community care charters. However, the government's demand for local community care charters – basically statements of quality (DoH, 1994) – was not accompanied by comparable stipulations for national standards, even though national voluntary organisations lobbied strongly during consultation over the 1994 document.

Care management

Care management offers a further instance of the incursion of managerialism into social care practice, replacing traditional social work skills with the management of care packages for individual users, linked to highly specified modes of assessment. The White Papers and the Audit Commission's 1992 report *Cascades of Change* situated the technique at the pinnacle of community care strategy.

American social services organisations developed 'case management' in the context of normally uncoordinated and independent hospitals or agencies. The method was imported into the UK in the 1970s and 1980s, emphasising the movement of mentally ill patients out of the hospitals and into the community. The concept influenced the Griffiths Report, the 1989 White Paper and the DoH Guidance. The central features of service diversity, adequate choice and the meeting of quality performance standards acceptable to users and carers, prioritised personal relationships and direct working with clients. Care management's prime functions comprise the identification of core tasks, setting achievement goals, assessing individual needs, care planning, plan implementation, monitoring and review. Doubts, though, remain with respect to the technique's effectiveness in the USA without adequate funding (Challis, 1994b; Payne, 1995).

The Kent project

Nevertheless, adaptations of the concept to care management in the UK have led to successful projects in client-orientated coordinated delivery of services, such as the pathbreaking Kent Community Care Scheme, much influenced by the University of Kent's Personal Social Services Research Unit (PSSRU). The project demonstrated that the greatest cost savings in community care are achievable by concentrating on those people with 'lower' levels of need and most likely to end up in residential care without the necessary home care support (Payne, 1995; Davies and Challis, 1986). Other care management projects were conducted in the 1980s and 1990s with older people, including the Gateshead Scheme, the Darlington Project, the EPIC Project in Scotland (Bland, 1994a), the Gloucester Project and projects in mental health (see Challis, 1994a, for a full review). A special 'care programme' approach operates for patients of consultant psychiatrists, with the purpose of closely involving patients and carers in preparation of care programmes and cooperation with nurses, GPs, social workers and other professionals. As we shall see, success has been very limited in this last sphere, but a number of the projects have encountered implementation problems.

Assessment

Client assessment is essential to the process of care management. Assessment, which falls very much under the jurisdiction of social work and constitutes a test of eligibility for care, requires various types of information such as social and ethnic background, abilities and lifestyle, personal history, carers' needs, housing and financial situation (Payne, 1995). But assessment of needs is inherently complex and definition of needs is difficult; final decisions may well depend upon the kind of information collected relating to a client's individual profile. As observed by Payne, 'the post-Griffiths community care model is inherently a *deficit* model of need', where the cause of a difficulty has to be defined as tightly as possible (ibid. p. 98).

While the assessment process should be viewed as a means of sensitising the manager to the users' own perspective of what services are necessary, local authority social services may use it for 'weeding out' or 'screening' those who are low down on the list, that is, it becomes, in effect, a rationing service. Also, the assessment process does not allow the full expression of actual needs but only those the local authority feels able to meet. Care management is already resource-driven at the assessment stage and weighted towards legitimating the bureaucratic decisions (Cornwell, 1992; Payne, 1995; Meredith, 1995).

Although rationing is a de facto function of the assessment process, it may be viewed as a channel for empowering service users and carers. Information gained from assessment, leading to unmet need, may be used for campaigning – a rather optimistic scenario. Or evidence of unmet need may be fed into the planning process. Yet many authorities, wary of legal challenge to any failure in meeting statutory duties, have shied away from formally recording the data. Other problems identified in the process include massive complications in the financial assessments and associated administration, disagreements between the assessors and users over the precise form of care outlined in the wake of assessment, and uneven GP involvement between areas. Most authorities seem to eschew the use of information gleaned from assessments in their future planning (Meredith, 1995).

Black African-Caribbean and other minority ethnic groups find the assessment stage unsatisfactory. The screening process rules out many people in Asian communities with 'hidden' needs who are further hampered by financial resourcing constraints (Law, 1996). Research in three local authorities (Begum, 1995) unearthed a host of difficulties for black minority ethnic group users, including obstacles to gaining an initial needs assessment and unclear eligibility criteria. The production of a viable 'care package' for a user erected additional hurdles such as culturally inappropriate or non-appropriate meals services (Law, 1996). (See Chapter 9 for discussion of other issues of minority ethnic groups and community care.)

Care managing and the social worker

With the culture of managerialism and cost effectiveness, it seemed almost self-evident that the job of care manager would not resemble the orthodox task of the social worker, even though the government never fully defined the role. After all, how particular to a profession is 'coordinating care'? Payne (1995) presents a robust case for the vital interpersonal skills of social workers in care management, although coordination and the devolvement of budgets entail greater management activity. Social work practice, he notes, lies at the heart of the American and Kent project models of care management.

Care managers are usually drawn from social services departments, although they may also include community health professionals (Bannerman and Robertson, 1996). However, information from recent case studies shows that care management has involved a complete change for 'front line' workers in their methods of working, coupled with distinctive secondary effects for social workers and their established mode of working. First, a greater proportion of management time is now devoted to highly dependent clients. Second, less time is available for counselling clients. The more practical tasks carried out in the past by social workers, but accorded lower status, are taking longer. Care managers pay more attention to administration of information collection on clients for assembling individual care packages than do social workers (Lewis and Glennerster, 1996). Although these new practices have created opportunities for a number of social workers, they have generated 'larger order' anxieties concerning organisational change and 'deskilling'.

Issues of implementation in care management

While the adoption of 'case management' in Britain has been viewed as innovative, the discussion on assessment procedures suggests that many problems arise in its implementation. The various case management pilots already mentioned did come up against existing or potential implementation snags. These included precise targeting of eligible user groups by the development of effective mechanisms, judging the best location of care management as between health and social care services, and the dangers of the purchaser:provider split leading to inappropriate care packages, and indeed the lack of a logical coherence in care management arrangements (Challis, 1994a).

Implementation of care management in Britain is a highly complicated task requiring proper resourcing which has not been forthcoming (the American community care projects have not been especially cost-effective). Care management tends to become administrative, not innovative or imaginative, and is overly bureaucratic. It deskills social work and discourages counselling. User and carers are likely to suffer rather than benefit (Sturges, 1996). A two-year monitoring project concluded that the drawbacks faced by care managers emanate from the contradictions implicit in the new community care policy's very objectives, such as the counterposing of competitiveness and innovation to stability and accountability, or of tight resources to the meeting of need. The context of the market acts as a dominant factor affecting the successful implementation of care management (Lewis *et al.*, 1995), besides the negative impacts on the workforce, as discussed below.

Changing organisations and social work pressures

Community care policies have dramatically altered the organisation of social care and services, closely affecting professional social workers. Managerialism and quasi-markets produce a marked effect upon their traditional skills' base, and educational and training requirements. Social workers' status is also threatened by the impending prospect of the disappearance of social services departments *per se* and the established functions of social work. But an accelerating speed of change compounded by inadequate resources aggravates occupational stress.

Global forces and social services organisations

The wider restructuring of the welfare state and local government constitutes the local context of social service reorganisation and social work practice. But it is also clear globalisation processes and post-Fordist tendencies (Chapter 1) have affected the redirection of funding from public to private welfare (Hoggett, 1994). The loss of a public sector ethic has arguably diminished caring professionals' power or influence over welfare policy and provision, and led to the deprofessionalisation of professional skills and the bureaucratisation of user involvement (Dominelli and Hoogvelt, 1996). Global market forces, accompanied by managerialist and budget-driven planning, serve to downgrade the status of holistic models and ethical caring in social work practice.

Senior managers in social services responsible for community care policy may well have enthusiatically embraced the managerialism of a global new public management movement (NPM) (Nixon, 1993). But it has tended to fragment and residualise social work in the course of its reconstruction, tantamount to 'the dismembering of social work' (Clarke, 1996).

Quality assurance and social work

Quality assurance (QA) is now applied in the public sector areas such as the health services, education and social services as a managerial tool derived from the post-Fordist restructuring or 'Japanisation' of manufacturing corporations (Ritchie, 1994). Yet while QA is a technique, some managers simultaneously treat it as a public management 'value' for promoting the management of power and control in organisations and the manipulation of change in an uncertain climate (James, 1992, 1994). Unsurprising, in the light of its business sector origins, the quality process implies a continuous inspection, measurement, evaluation and monitoring of services aimed at consumer satisfaction. One may contend that such monitoring is not necessarily a bad thing, but it is a constricting process which bears all the hallmarks of an 'assembly line' (Cassam and Gupta, 1992; Wing, 1992; Beazley, 1994; Meredith, 1995). It is also singularly inappropriate in community care, where service quality is awkward to measure and susceptible to diverse interpretation by purchasers, providers and users (Beazley, 1994).

The promotion of quality assurance, measurement and competencies may be taken as signifying the central 'value' of management control which has come to displace social work values and approaches rooted in medicine, psychiatry and therapy (Dominelli, 1996). The focus on discrete competencies for defining requisite skills serves as an ideological management technique control, since it fragments holistic judgement and challenges the autonomy of the critical reflective practitioner (Dominelli and Hoogvelt, 1996; Dominelli, 1996). Competence-led definitions of professional skills in community care minister to the quality assurance mechanisms of new public management in the contract culture, so that now the relationship between social worker and 'client' reflects technical arrangements and process-led manoeuvring for resources.

Social workers' conditions, occupational stress and community care

All of the changes noted above, along with the restrictions in staffing budgets, have produced extensive physical and emotional effects on social workers. Surveys and reports on serious stress among social workers multiply. Social workers have long suffered from occupational stress. However, the circumstances of community care's implementation through 'imposed change involving less secure pay and conditions with inadequate resources' are most liable to result in increased stress (Carpenter, 1994, p. 98) through the 'service trap'; workers strive to bridge a widening care gap, but worsen their own health and endure mounting professional frustration. Occupational stress research has found that social workers experience stress from organisational restructuring, including problems stemming from inadequate and inappropriate resources, demoralisation from time pressures and paperwork overload, emotional and physical exhaustion, irritability and muscular tension (Bradley and Sutherland, 1995; Caughey, 1996). Another study of practitioners' experiences under the new community care concluded that 'almost all workers now report levels of stress from workloads that have increased to the point that they have little time, energy or enthusiasm to plan to advance their training and their careers' (Hadley and Clough, 1996, p. 189). Case studies document rising frustrations on the part of social workers-cum-care managers as direct work with clients shrinks, while the paper work has burgeoned since the implementation of community care (Francis, 1996b).

The rapid reorientation from traditional social work to care management in community care has taken its personal toll. But some social work analysts and practitioners argue that a crucial way forward lies in effective multidisciplinary training for social workers which incorporates up-to-date community care practice, and in developing management skills (Payne, 1995). Competencies dominate the employer-led training of social workers (Brown, 1994). Previous commitments to equal opportunities and anti-racism were squeezed out of social work education (CCETSW, 1995), reflecting the ideological nature of managerialism and its anti-professional construction in community care and the new social services (Chapter 1). Obedience to markets, training for management skills and an implicitly ideological anti-intellectualism pose real threats to the continuation of any real social work education (Jones, 1996).

The shifting organisation of social services, in sum, represents an amalgam of global restructuring processes, New Right social policy and managerialist policy directives which has splintered the social work profession. Management is invested with the stature of 'value' arguably antithetical to the activity of social care. Community care policy's incorporation of consumerism has meant extensive organisational restructuring and related stress among the social care workforce. While elements of this occupational stress may be rectified by systematic training, the *nature* of such retraining is deeply ideological in its devaluation of critical thought.

Comparative social care developments

The literature on social care services in comparative social policy research is rather thin (Anttonen and Sipila, 1996; Alber, 1995). Insofar as the state is concerned, delivery of community care in the United States is of a residual nature. As we have seen in Chapter 3, health care exhibits a strong market orientation, steered by overt capitalist values. Self-help groups and the voluntary sector play a big role; social agencies are few, social care being dominated by the institutions of Medicare and Medicaid (Tester, 1996a).

European economies, closer to the British system, have implemented similar types of restructuring in a distinct movement towards welfare pluralism. For example, Italy and France experienced more decentralisation, and greater consumer participation and choice, as well as adopting care management techniques and individualised 'care package' delivery in the 1980s. These new departures may be seen as especially radical for Italy, recognised for its strong reliance on family care and the church (Lorenz, 1994).

The Netherlands is replacing institutional care with community care, not least due to the strong ideological policy influences from the political New Right, emphasising an enhanced role for the market. Anxieties have mounted over the difficulties of coordinating health and welfare services, paralleling the British situation. Problems of health and social care services coordination are experienced even in Denmark, where home care organisation is considered highly successful (Means and Smith, 1994).

The thrust of Germany's community care lies in its social insurance system (now a major theme of British social policy debate). Compulsory insurance has been introduced, but social support services, on the other hand, are less developed. As in Britain's case, informal caring is most significant, usually provided by women:

more than 80 per cent of Germany's infirm elderly and chronically ill people are cared for by their daughter or daughter-in-law (Ginsburg, 1992).

Spain's welfare state is minimalist, and problems exist in coordinating personal social services and supplying care evenly, not least because of pressures to reduce public spending. Services have been decentralised, but the extent of privatisation has been less marked (George and Taylor-Gooby, 1996).

As in Britain, Sweden's Social Democrats moved towards the adoption of community care through the 1980s. Many social institutions were closed, while government overhauled elderly persons' care at the turn of the decade. Communes became responsible for all residential provision for old persons. The new system involved the transfer of a number of services from health care authorities to county councils. The country's new right-wing government of 1992, however, promoted more private, voluntary and cooperative care (Gould, 1996).

The European Union and community care

European Union policies play only a limited part in community care social care policies. Yet no European programmes are specifically geared towards supporting the provision of social care services (Swithibank, 1996). The European Social Fund (ESF) is a prime source of finance for groups such as people with mental health problems, but the Fund has huge drawbacks. In the first place, it tends not to assist the most vulnerable and dependent. Second, it is extremely slow in advancing the cash, which hits small organisations (Swithibank, 1996) and can spell disaster for voluntary groups (Snell, 1996).

European legislation plus the Community Charter indicate provisions for older and disabled people. The Union places the onus on the member states to guarantee minimum levels of subsistence, aiming to minimise disparities in spending on care for older and disabled people (Hantrais, 1995). An Observatory on Ageing and Older People was instituted in the 1990s, concentrating on four areas including health and social care, while a 1994 White Paper on European social policy introduced measures for the elimination of discrimination against disabled people (Hantrais, 1995).

Financing of social care

Cost control seems to drive most of the western capitalist economies towards the adoption of community care systems which minimise reliance on expensive institutional social care, a sure sign that the post-Thatcherite climate is no longer exclusive to Britain (Paul, 1996). This means the siphoning of funds out of acute and institutional modes of care delivery and into domiciliary and community care for chronically ill and disabled persons (Tester, 1996a).

The introduction of care insurance, as in Germany, France and Italy, mirrors the ideological transformation from dependence on state provision to the principle of individual and family responsibility. Such a strategy, in effect, strengthens the emphasis on dual welfare provision and the associated creation of an insurance–assistance divide between those who are able to insure themselves and those who must turn to marginalised and stigmatised services funded through state social assistance mechanisms (Tester, 1996a).

Pluralism, decentralisation and marketisation are not just specific to community care policies in Britain, then, but dovetail with economic global change and the spread of New Right ideologies; economies motivated to reduce overall care costs are withdrawing resources from state institutional care, while private and 'mixed' social insurance schemes are growing in importance.

Conclusion

New community care policies have reshaped health and social care delivery within the new policy paradigm. Traditional institutional models of care cease to hold the same meaning, yet domestic caring becomes pivotal to government policy. Legislation has altered local authority functions and transferred the financial burdens from central government to the localities. All this is happening against an environment of global economic restructuring, dominant managerialist values and the predominance of market relationships.

Local authorities' new enabling role reflects the welfare mix which effectively reduces local state powers, but it is questionable as to whether entrepreneurialism and the purchaser:provider split are compatible with user participation. The enhanced role of the independent sector reflects social policy's reorientation to civil society, yet the contract culture threatens the future of voluntary bodies in the absence of stable funding. Imperatives for planning community care occasion dual effects, in that they emphasise the necessity for improved collaboration and precise information, while exposing the paucity of existing collaboration, 'consumer' involvement and the actual complexities of the system. New care management techniques may spotlight the need for individually informed care and detailed assessment, but successful implementation demands proper resourcing. Organisational restructuring not only affects users, but has resulted in stress, uncertainty and professional devaluation among social workers. Finally, the new community care model is by no means an exclusively British phenomenon; the New Right policy paradigm of care market efficiency is common to a number of other Western capitalist economies, despite the low profile adopted by the European Union's social policy institutions. In Part II of this book, we will scrutinise more closely the impacts of community care policies upon discrete user groups, and explore wider social policy issues of equity, anti-discrimination and citizenship.

Further reading

GOSTRICK, C., DAVIES, B., LAWSON, R. and SALTER, C. (1997) *From Vision To Reality In Community Care: Changing direction at the local level*, Aldershot: Arena. Evaluation of community care strategy, management and implementation over ten years, using primary case studies.

MANDELSTAM, M. with SCHWER, B. (1995) *Community Care Practice and the Law*, London: Jessica Kingsley. An indispensable reference work.

HANVEY, C. and PHILPOT, T. (eds) (1996) *Sweet Charity: The role and workings of voluntary organisations*, London: Routledge. Contributors examine the shifting functions of the voluntary sector in the new contract culture.

GEORGE, V. and TAYLOR-GOOBY, P. (eds) (1996) *European Welfare Policy: Squaring the welfare circle*, London: Macmillan. Specialists assessing broad welfare provision in seven European economies.

PART II

USER GROUPS AND COMMUNITY CARE

5

ELDERLY PERSONS AND COMMUNITY CARE

Introduction

Usually when we refer to old age, we are dealing with the final stage (or stages) of life. Life for older people poses a number of issues not encountered by young people. However, chronological age is not necessarily the defining element for problems in old age; nor is the latter a single undifferentiated age set. But older people have traditionally been treated as if this *were* the case. A whole set of attitudes, a 'way of seeing', has contributed to the shaping of social policy.

Old age as a discrete stage in the life process is a modern phenomenon, in that the proportion of retired people has grown considerably during this century. State pensions have become institutionalised, while retirement has become the 'norm' rather than the exception (Pilcher, 1995). On the one hand, such trends may be perceived as endowing older people with enhanced status (Johnson, 1989). On the other hand, social policy analysts such as Townsend (1981) suggest that these developments contribute to the structuring of dependency in modern British society. To this extent, the greater demographic significance of older people has been interpreted as a social problem for policy makers and society at large, stemming from notions of old people as burden, a modified type of race or class discrimination which deals in stereotypes of old age in the form of ageism (Bornat *et al.*, 1985; McEwen, 1990).

But the condition of older people cannot be characterised by monolithic features. It does indeed depend upon other factors to do with social class, ethnicity, gender and disability. Hence, talk of the 'elderly' is misguided, as though old people constitute an undifferentiated mass. As we shall see in this chapter, the issues of caring for old people, and the formulated strategies, are tightly bound to ideological constructions of their particular social importance.

The chapter will discuss in greater detail the global and national demographic trends in relation to older people, the ideological constructions which bear upon attitudes and policies, the areas of state social policy which have affected older people, specific issues in current community care for old persons, the particular economic difficulties and policies affecting these groups, and comparative issues.

Demographic trends and ageing

The demography of ageing is pertinent at a number of spatial scales – global and regional, in Western Europe, Third World countries, and in Britain. In each case, the ageing population has grown relatively and absolutely, a trend bringing in its wake important changes in family structure. During the present century the proportion of people aged 60 and over has increased in the economically 'advanced' industrialised nations due to the declining birth rate and a general improvement in life expectancy (Bond *et al.*, 1993; Sen, 1994). In Western Europe the proportion in the 60-plus age group grew from 6 per cent in 1901 to 18 per cent in 1991, a considerable section of the the total population (Hugman, 1994; Hughes, B., 1995; Hantrais, 1995). The same trends have operated in absolute terms. For example, the number of older people rose from some 2 million to 10.5 million in Britain between 1901 and 1991.

Even more significant changes are occurring within the band of the 60-plus age group. There are expected to be 2.9 million people of 75 or older by the year 2025, indicating an ageing of the older population, producing a division between 'young old' and 'older old' , even though many older people are now enjoying their 'Third Age' (Laslett, 1996). But care policies tend to ignore crucial gender differences in caring needs, as we shall see, because of deeply embedded ideological assumptions of gender roles and the social division of labour.

With respect to ethnic differences, the ageing structure of minority ethnic groups in Britain does not replicate that of the white population. Much lower proportions among minority ethnic groups are of pensionable age (3–5 per cent, as against 19 per cent) than in the white population, although this varies between minority ethnic groups. The West Indian proportion tends to be higher than for Asians (Owen, 1995). Nevertheless, the numbers of 'old old' among the minority ethnic groups have increased in the 1990s, demanding similar levels of urgency for caring in the future (Patel, 1993). By the year 2000 there will have been a 400–500 per cent increase in the size of the pensionable age group (Blakemore and Boneham, 1994).

Changes in the family structure

Economic, technological, demographic, legal, and ideological changes have influenced the formation of families over the past century (Jerrome, 1993). Demographic trends, including reduced family size and marriage at a younger age, have narrowed the gap between generations. The greater numbers of females in the work-force have extended their own work career horizons, thereby altering perceptions of their expected role within the family household. Divorce legislation has facilitated more fluid and open-ended, divided family structures that blur the historical lines of 'obligation' to care for the earlier generations. Ideologically, the Conservative Government's promotion of traditional family values and the nuclear family structure (in the formal political rhetoric) placed the emphasis for community care upon the family, although the actual family patterns and belief systems vis-à-vis social living arrangements run counter to such ideology. Each of these changes affects the kind of support offered within families, namely, economic support, accommodation, personal care, practical support, and emotional and moral support (Finch, 1989). In the light of policy which equates community with family care, the demographic and economic shifts would suggest that the social support services will be only minimal; the need for intensive care is constantly growing at a time when the number offering intensive care is declining (Qureshi, 1996). Such trends are compounded by ageist attitudes, as discussed below.

Ageing, ideology and discrimination

The status of old age in the West has not been an elevated one either historically or culturally, thus bearing upon policy and practical interventions. According to the *Encyclopaedia of Ageing*, ageism is defined as 'a process of systematic stereotyping of, and discrimination against, people because they are old, just as racism and sexism accomplish this for skin colour and gender' (Butler, 1987, p. 22). Ageism may be seen as an attitude (ideology) which treats old people as an undifferentiated mass, assigns stereotypes to their behaviour and projects insulting images which undercut their sense of personal worth and value (Scrutton, 1990). This process interacts with other sets of ideological 'othering' such as racism, sexism and disablism in shaping economic and social policies and the personal experiences of old people (Biggs, 1993).

However, ageism applies to us *all*, irrespective of age. We each experience constraints: 'The chronology of ageing becomes the hierarchy of ageism' (Itzen, 1986, p. 114). Legislative discrimination and exclusion is a form of ageist discrimination comparable to other discriminatory forms accompanying personal insult (Bytheway and Johnson, 1990). Hughes (Hughes, B., 1995) conceptualises the process of the social construction of ageing and ageism as produced by a society's economic structure, political values, cultural heritage, historical legacy and social attitudes; this construction informs central and local policies and quasi-governmental agencies, personal and professional interactions, and older people's situation. Gerontology's status within the medical profession is low, akin to that of 'elderly' care teams in social services' departments, sustaining poor levels of training and subject to low allocation of resources (ibid.).

Ageism, racism and sexism

Ageism for women combines with sexism to form a double bind of discrimination: the double standard of ageing, which differentiates older women's treatment from that of men (Arber and Ginn, 1995). If females break out of their allotted roles (reproduction and caring) during their lives, then they suffer in old age through job discrimination and poor income support entitlements (Arber and Ginn, 1991).

Older black people and Asians are similarly marginalised and devalued in job markets and within other social contexts under capitalism. The evidence is equivocal as to whether black and Asian elders in deprived inner-city areas are any more deprived than poorer older whites whose life situations are spiralling downwards and whose social support is almost non-existent. Clearly, the complexity of ageism must also encompass the effects of social class (Blakemore and Boneham, 1994). Nevertheless, members of minority ethnic groups *qua* minorities face discrimination and harassment over their rights of citizenship, employment, health and welfare service provision and standards of accommodation (Fennell *et al.*, 1988; Ahmad, 1996).

Ageism, discrimination and disablism

Attitudes towards people with disabilities have been narrow and limiting; hence, as we shall discuss in Chapter 6, older people with disabilities certainly feel the impacts of disablism which serve to marginalise them from everyday social activities and opportunities (Zarb and Oliver, 1992). Not much research, however, has been conducted on the dual impact of ageism and disablism. Many disabled people discover similarities in their objective situation as they grow older (Zarb, 1993). Exactly how individual disabled people deal with ageing is again dependent on other variables such as class, gender and race. Because of their earlier struggles to create their own identity and independence, many older women place more weight than males on maintenance of their independence in old age. Again, not much research deals with ethnic differences on ageing with a disability, although the combination of discriminatory factors leads to a cumulative disadvantage – 'triple jeopardy' in the receipt of health and social services (Norman, 1985; Begum, 1992; Patel, 1993; Blakemore and Boneham, 1994). The danger of such concepts, though, is that they assume a homogeneity among these distinct groups that does not really exist (Stuart, 1992, 1996).

Elder abuse

The widespread nature of discrimination has led to the notable neglect of older people, especially when frail and highly dependent, which frequently culminates in abuse. The publicity has

115

usually been directed at those in residential institutions. Cases have revealed residents illegally deprived of money, physical and sexual assault, and queuing naked for a bath (Scrutton, 1990).

A greater public and professional awareness of elder abuse occurs in Canada and the United States, where many more resources have been devoted to researching and formulating policy than in Britain (Ogg and Munn-Giddings, 1993). Nevertheless, the research has not managed to completely integrate the important gender dimension of elder abuse, given the evidence that in society so much violence and abuse is directed against females, linked to the power nexus and the 'othering' of women in the wider patriarchal society (see Margaret Forster's novel *Has He Had Enough to Eat?*).

The approach to the problem stems from a distinctly familialist ideology. Many explanations have focused on elder abuse in terms of carer stress or family pathology (Bennet and Kingston, 1993). However, argues Whittaker, elder abuse is more complicated than this, and cannot be solved by policies simply founded on support for carers. Proper analysis of elder abuse should take into account older women's social structural position in this society, and their resources for resisting abusive behaviour within the family (Whittaker, 1995).

Health policy and older people

The main aspects of modern British social policy addressing the needs and issues of older people ostensibly fall into the categories of the changing health policies discussed in Chapter 3, and the areas of social care until recently seen as distinct and governed largely by the 1948 National Assistance Act. With 'Working For Patients' and the promotion of GP funded practices, research has pointed towards a relative failure to follow up contacts with elderly people after check-up, in spite of the requirement to offer older persons a home visit. The proposals have favoured the wealthier practices, an implicit disadvantage for most older people. The shift from single doctor to group practices and health centres has facilitated the provision of primary health care in more purpose-built and comfortable premises, and access for older people to nurses on a regular basis. Nevertheless, the rationalising of practices usually entails longer travel distances for elderly people without adequate transport. Formalised appointments procedures disadvantage the many elderly non-telephone users and devalue personalised medical service. Some lone GP practices in inner-city areas are in 'lock-up' premises and less accessible (Tinker, 1992). A series of evaluation studies on the impacts of new health policies for older people found greater numbers waiting for hospital treatment; there was no real change in choice of hospital, or quality of service, although health assessments have increased in line with the modifications to GP contracts (Jones *et al.*, 1993).

Notwithstanding the low volume of research, it is evident that black elders have been ill-served by the health services (Patel, 1993). The quality of service from GPs has been uncertain: for instance, poor services for dealing with hearing problems. In spite of the existence of maternity or child health services, there is no known scheme involving health visitors for elderly people among the minority ethnic groups (Pharoah and Redmond, 1991). Such inadequacies in health service provision for black elders may be explained (in similar fashion for black and Asian communities as a whole – see Chapter 9) by a series of racisms: institutional and individual racism and internal 'colonialism' (Patel, 1993). Structural changes in primary health care and GP services, then, mean increased access difficulties and no real expansion in choice, while services for minority ethnic groups remain substandard. But what of social care services?

Social care, personal services and social policy

As we have already seen, the initiation of a comprehensive postwar welfare state in Britain meant a substantial difference for social care of the population, and a more consistent role was accorded state intervention by social services. The National Assistance Act 1948, dealing with the provision of residential care as distinct from health care, is considered a radical turning point in recognition of the social needs of elderly people (see Chapter 2). The Act imposed duties on local authorities to provide such homes, and further local authority duties included the provision of domiciliary support, although the responsibilities were minimal relative to those for residential care.

Domiciliary care

Surveys indicate that the bulk of domiciliary services tend to be utilised by those over 75 years of age, by females and those people living on their own (Office of Population Census Statistics, 1989; Tinker, 1992). The proportion of people aged 65 years and over in receipt of home help has generally stayed at 9 per cent. But unmet need remains, regardless of the upgrading of the community care policy. The home help service has been rather restrictive and 'spread too thinly'; elderly people are unlikely to receive assistance with traditional home help duties like shopping or cleaning unless they also demonstrate more intensive needs (Tinker, 1992, p. 149).

Day care services are provided outside of the old person's home, relying on heavy input from voluntary services, and meet a number of needs, including physical, emotional, recreational and educational, and also encompass respite care for carers engaged in evening or night care.

Residential care

Numbers in residential care aged 65 and over increased from 152,897 in 1979 to 232,527 in 1989, but the increase in private residential homes was more dramatic (from 29,095 to 111,391) because of the availability of a board and lodging allowance paid by DHSS. The new private and voluntary homes are subject to registration and inspection under the Residential Homes Act 1980 and the Registered Homes Act 1984 (Tinker, 1992).

However, whether many older people have been appropriately placed in residential care is a contentious matter. Some may have been allocated there because of a lack of suitable housing. And a growing number of much older, frail and confused people are being admitted to residential homes when they clearly need nursing care (Tinker, 1992). On the other hand, the Wagner Report, *Residential Care: A positive choice*, following in the wake of the1988 Griffiths' Report, placed emphasis on the positive aspects to residential care. It argued that older people should not be forced to move because of changing needs, and also called for enhanced choice and rights within residential care and a set of principles for improved quality. A Court of Appeal ruling on Sefton Council's responsibilities has proved much in favour of elderly people with limited incomes, ensuring that local authorities are bound to pay for long-term care in residential homes for residents with less than £10,000 in savings (*Guardian*, 1 August 1997).

The role of the voluntary sector for elderly persons

Voluntary bodies or organisations (Chapter 4) with respect to older people have served a number of functions: provision of homes and financial assistance to elderly people living in poverty or who are disabled (e.g. Rowntree Trust); raising funds (e.g. Help the Aged); visiting older people (e.g. churches); funding research on older people (e.g. Nuffield). But what are the particular issues for old people arising from the operation of voluntary bodies? First is the problem of variability in standards, which is related to social-class differences between older people (Tinker, 1997). Second, the voluntary organisations' lines of responsibility are not always clear; voluntary bodies often serve a small self-selected group and are not accountable to the wider network of old people. Third, the operation of three major national voluntary bodies (Help the Aged, Age Concern, and Centre for Policy on Ageing) leads to serious voluntary group duplication. Fourth, the 'charity image' lingers on for old people. However, this is not something specific to voluntary bodies but applies to such processes as the perceived stigma in claiming statutory benefits (Tinker, 1992). The question of resources is important, seeing as the independence of such bodies depends more than ever on the money they are able to raise in line with their new duties under community care legislation.

Community care policies and caring for older people

The 1990 NHS and Community Care Act gave local authorities the major responsibility for coordination and producing care assessments for older people. Local authorities were impelled to carry out comprehensive assessment of needs for anyone where it was felt necessary. This procedure is viewed as crucial for determining decisions at the level of resources and funding, plus the means whereby central principles such as choice and user and carer participation are actually implemented (Hughes, B., 1995). The change from state-administered residential homes to non-state forms of provision 'in the community' or the individual home, has tended to 'privatise' much of the care for elderly persons. Emphasis upon 'mixed' packages of care for old people would seem to have reduced the complexity arising from the involvement of different authorities and agencies in care delivery. However, the purchaser: provider distinction leads to conflicts (Chapters 3 and 4) between health and social care organisations as to who pays for long-term care of elderly people. The frequently posed question is: 'Where does free NHS care end and means-tested social care begin?' Cervi (1996) argues that the problem of the care of elderly people is 'bogged down in this structural divide', not unrelated to the fact that NHS resources are committed to the acute sector, yet community services and joint initiatives with local authorities are undervalued and underresourced. Whereas the number of cooperative initiatives for people with mental health and learning difficulties is growing, this has not been so with services for elderly people (Cervi, 1996).

Although most old people are affected by this realignment to the 'community', it is obvious that elderly women are more disadvantaged; they must rely more on the 'community' and the state, given the differences in household care and financial independence. Twice as many elderly women as men require care or support to remain in the community. Fourteen per cent of elderly women are severely disabled, as compared with 7 per cent of men. In a replication of traditional social attitudes *vis-à-vis* the domestic division of labour, men are more likely as of right to enjoy access to privileged caring resources. Lone elderly women more regularly lack material resources and also suffer more from poor health than do their male counterparts (Arber and Ginn, 1991). Personal finance, as discussed below, is clearly a major problem for elderly people.

Community care, elderly people and financial difficulties

The relocation from residential to community-based care does pose a number of problems for elderly persons. Access to essential resources such as material and financial health and access to caring resources will influence how effectively older persons' needs will be met while also attempting to ensure a level of independence (Arber and Ginn, 1991). Without such personal resources, older people must either look to their own household, the community or the state. The ability of older people to benefit from community care is anchored to their financial situation, but community care policies have been insufficiently related to other policies, which are either too weak to counter people's financial vulnerability or, in effect, exacerbate it.

Class, retirement and security

Once retired, access to employment is cut off for many older people due to ageist attitudes by employers, making retirement a financially insecure condition. Living in the community becomes a hardship in the absence of adequate material resources (McEwen, 1990). Inequalities based on economic class experienced during employment in early life reproduce themselves in old age. Those working in manual and low-paid occupations experience poor benefits and a declining standard of living later in life. The 1995 Pensions Act has weakened the state earnings-related pension (SERPS) by reducing protection for those who cannot afford private coverage (Oppenheim and Harker, 1996). Discrimination within the social security system militates against elderly persons, especially those who are disabled, in that males aged 60-plus and females aged 55-plus have not received invalidity allowance (Walker, 1990, p. 66). An estimated 220,000 people lost out because of benefits changes in 1995 (Oppenheim and Harker, 1996, pp. 60–1). One may measure this financial insecurity against the expectations of older people financing their own care. Such barriers to satisfactory community care illustrate the narrow vision of social policies such as for pensions, housing and care services, formulated in isolation (Baldwin, 1994).

Poverty, ageing and gender

Pensioners remain in the high risk poverty categories at the closing of the twentieth century. Twenty-six per cent of pensioner couples and 35 per cent of predominantly female single pensioners are living in poverty (Oppenheim and Harker, 1996, p. 36). The financial position of older women is particularly serious. They receive less from occupational pensions, state entitlements are lost from the years of caring, and care allowances yield scant compensation for the missed earnings (Baldwin, 1994). Community care policies produce severe personal financial impacts. Heavy reliance on informal and unpaid care, coupled with the vagaries of the social security system, leads to inadequate incomes for many elderly and disabled females, and a huge loss of earnings and benefits, invariably presaging poverty for their own old age (Glendinning, 1992). Once again, disjointed policy making, whereby employment, social security and community care policies develop independently of each other, becomes part of the problem.

Poverty appears to be the central financial problem facing older females with minimal income, compounded by class position, racial discrimination and ageism in the society at large. Women, comprising some 65 per cent of the elderly population, are much more likely than men to be poor pensioners. More than five times as many depend on income support (Oppeheim and Harker, 1996, p. 61). Women's poor pension position, argue Ginn and Arber (1994) is largely attributable to the patriarchy of the Beveridge Plan and the British government's boost of occupational pensions (unlike in other European societies) which fail to meet women's needs. Hence, the suggestion that pension and retirement schemes should be completely accountable to sex discrimination legislation (Groves, 1992).

Poverty, ethnicity and old age

Information is seriously lacking on the older minority ethnic population (Hughes, B., 1995). 'Ethnicity' has been marginalised from social security policy research, due to the paucity of DSS funding for such research, and the lack of ethnic monitoring systems in key agencies (Craig, 1996; Craig and Rai, 1996). Much of the work on older groups has to be speculative. The older population constitutes a much smaller proportion (3 per cent of minority ethnic groups) than they do among the white UK population (17 per cent). However, whereas minority ethnic elders may enjoy greater access to informal carers, their low incomes and longer periods spent in unemployment denote a high probability that pensioners from minority ethnic groups will suffer poorer access to state and occupational pensions and other contributory benefits. This is made worse by visits home to maintain family links, which lead to breaks in pension contributions and a lower retirement pension. Yet the community care legislation made almost no reference to caring for minority ethnic group elders (Craig and Rai, 1996; Oppenheim and Harker, 1996).

Clearly, the ability of old people to survive in the community is highly dependent on their earlier economic class position and their consequent entitlements upon retirement, to the point where elderly people fall into the poverty category.

Funding long-term care

Funding long-term care has become particularly important, with the requirements for social services and health authorities to produce community plan agreements on continuing care, and the interrelated responsibilities of health and social services (Hancock, 1995). Many clients are elderly people, usually female and in possession of few resources, usually on the poverty line and growing in numbers. The central government had forged no strategy for funding until the approach of the 1997 General Election; local authorities are attempting to shunt clients back to the health authorities or are leaving the greater numbers of dependent elderly people with substandard care because of cash shortage. The budgetary constraints have led to elderly persons with high levels of disability being cared for in residential homes without suitable facilities or staffing arrangements, instead of receiving nursing home care. Similarly, many elderly people placed in nursing or residential homes should really be in receipt of hospital care (O'Kell, 1996).

Sensing in 1996 the pressures of the impending General Election, the Conservative Government trawled for new ideas from policy institutes and academies (*The Times*, 8 May 1996). The House of Commons Select Committee called for a new type of social insurance payment to replace a compulsory universal welfare state levy, which left some payment up to the individual. The funding of health care and social care elements in long-term care was to be kept separate (Professional Social Work, 1996). This divorce of health and social care funding was challenged by the Joseph Rowntree Foundation's major report in September, 1996. Rowntree proposed collective provision on the German social insurance scheme model, with all employed people paying an income-related amount. Age Concern was also lobbying for the government to increase the level of the 'preserved rights' income support, so that it would be able to meet care costs in full. The clear trend in all such proposals was the advocacy of 'partnership' between the world of insurance and social policy makers in government (*Guardian*, 14 September 1996; *Guardian*, 12 March 1997; Kohler, 1996).

Empowerment, community care and elderly persons

Given the philosophy of community care legislation, particularly with respect to the accountability and participation of clients, how have the older client groups fared? It is relevant to raise such queries of elderly people, since the 1989 White Paper 'Caring For People' posited the need for stimulating choice for service users as a key reason for transformations in community care. The DHSS Inspectorate (1991) announced the empowerment of users and carers as the rationale for the 1990 health and social care re-organisation (cited in Means and Lart, 1994).

Means and Lart (1994) present a ladder of empowerment scaling degrees of power conferred on users, from those having the authority to take decisions down to simply being given information about decisions already made. In between lie degrees of empowerment where users possess the authority for taking *some* decisions; an opportunity for *influencing* decisions; where their views are *sought* before decisions are made; and where decisions are publicised and explained before implementation.

A survey of community care plans produced by four statutory social services authorities (Hammersmith and Fulham, St Helens, Oxfordshire and Devon) in the early 1990s revealed the weak involvement of older users of community care in user groups, as compared with other user groups. They had enjoyed little opportunity to comment on the local community care strategy (Hoyes and Lart, 1992). Another early study (Allen *et al.*, 1992) found that elderly people were conceded little voice or influence over the level of services they received. What confuses matters is the particular reluctance of older persons to be critical (Hoyes and Means, 1991). But the danger remains of stereotyping older women – despite older people's wide range of circumstances nowadays and their generally improved health – and older people suffering from senile dementia.

Involvement of minority ethnic groups in consultation is unimpressive. Gandhi (1996) describes an Open Space Forum funded project in Liverpool. Despite open participation by elderly people, including those from minority ethnic communities, the latter encountered barriers to communication. Gandhi concludes that professionals 'need to improve relationships with ethnic minority groups especially and must encourage greater openness and trust between senior management, front-line workers, service users and carers' (ibid. p. 13).

But older people in general are certainly capable of mobilisation. Social movements among older people have developed largely in Australia and America. The National Pensioners' Convention (NPC) acts as the key umbrella organisation for pensioners' movements in the UK. Aimed at achieving equality of basic living standards across Europe and run by volunteers, the movement campaigns on issues including care in the community and countering ageism (Thain, 1995).

As part of the wider movement, pensioners' forums in Britain go back to the 1930s, initially focusing on economic issues but more recently encompassing community care policy. The growth of forums in particular has been motivated by the demand for a local voice which has hardly been met by the more distant, politically conscious national campaigning. Such forums have offered a channel for older people's voices to be heard within the local authority decision-making framework (Carter and Nash, 1995).

Although there are more retired women than men, the former are underrepresented in leadership roles. This is also the case for older people from minority ethnic groups (Carter and Nash, 1995). Nevertheless, the Older Women's Project has grown out of the broad movement, mobilising around anti-ageism, poor health, and poverty among older women; this, in turn, has stimulated older Caribbean women to organise around specific types of sickness. The Project (under the banner of the London based AGLOW) has also taken up the issue of slack formal support for older women carers whose voice has traditionally remained mute (Curtis, 1995). Other relatively successful political campaigns include that of the Action on Elder Abuse pressure group which has exerted an impact by ensuring that discussion of the practice is granted a higher profile on the public policy agenda (Slater, 1995).

Comparative policies and community care for elderly people

How has community care worked for elderly people in other countries? New methods for financing care have operated in a number of economies with varying results since the 1980s. The quality of pensions is correlated with the particular political and ideological framework in social policy making (Esping-Anderson, 1990; Mishra, 1990; Ginsburg, 1992). For example, the French system is based upon the solidarity principle (a guaranteed income plus voluntary schemes), while the American residualist pension system offers a low state pension but more significant private occupational pensions. Britain too operates a residual system with its flat-rate universal basic pension and a large occupational pension sector. Access to the pensions and benefits system also depends on older persons' differentiated position in terms of gender, 'race', class and geographical location: for example, in the case of the unequally provided Southern and Northern Italians; those in the states of the new federated Germany as opposed to the old (Tester, 1996a); and differences between federated states as in Australia (Gibson, 1996). Across the European nations, and in the USA, women are greatly disadvantaged by pensions systems which depend on a husband's contributions. In France, Germany, the Netherlands and the USA, older people from minority ethnic groups have lost out on pension benefits and are thus vulnerable to poverty. Although the 'social democratic' Netherlands offers the most substantial benefits for older males and females, in contrast to the minimal entitlements of the 'liberal' regimes of Britain and USA, the financing of long-term care for dependent elderly persons nevertheless poses a challenge for all systems.

Domiciliary and day care

Domiciliary care has been provided for a long time in European Union countries and Scandinavia, but is of more recent origin in the southern economies of Greece, Spain and Portugal. The medical–social divide has played a major role in influencing older people and their carers (Alber, 1993). Tester (1996a, p. 99) suggests that medical incentives in the funding system mean that 'services are provided on a medical model designed to cure rather than a social model geared to care for frail older people with long-term needs'. Some form of day care is available in most of the European states, but hospital day care is usually for rehabilitation in countries like France, Italy, Denmark and the UK (Hugman, 1994). Success in the provision of such care for older people depends on coordination between health and social care. While policy seems to be orientated towards assessment of individual needs in the 1990s, other areas such as non-statutory provision elicit fragmentation and widening inequalities in access to services.

Informal and formal caring

Reflecting the strains upon informal family care in Britain, EU countries have experienced a shrinkage in availability of female carers, due to increased female actvity rates in the job market. But unlike Denmark, a number of states have denied the state's responsibility for caring for older people. Family relatives in Germany, Italy and France have had to contribute to domiciliary and residential services on a means-tested basis.

A comparative analysis of six countries (Finland, Sweden, Italy, Germany, France and Ireland) underlines the dangers and complications of payments for informal care, especially where used to recruit new carers rather than to supply longer-term care and avoid institutionalised care. Care allowances are also devoted to basics (food and heating) instead of bona fide care in the absence of viable social security payments (Glendinning and McLaughlin, 1993).

Gender, 'race', and class inequalities

As noted above, uneven access to community care services affects elderly persons' care in different countries. Gender differentials are important, as illustrated by studies in Germany, Finland, Sweden, Denmark and Norway, where male carers receive greater care support, with the exception of Denmark (Siim, 1990; Waerness, 1990; Hugman, 1994). Women of all ages are likely to be caring for an older person in Germany, Italy, Greece, Sweden, Denmark and France. Men are the most likely to be elderly carers looking after partners in Britain and the Netherlands.

Issues of racial inequalities have hardly been addressed in European countries, owing to the currently low proportions of ethnic minority elders (and of course the respective colonialist racist histories) (Hugman, 1994). European research on social-class disadvantages in access to community care for older people based on social class has reinforced the notion that social advantages assist middle and upper classes. For example, open-care centres in Greece are used more frequently by the more affluent. Germany has transferred direct costs to older people, while social class differentiates the extent of community care received by older people in Italy (Hugman, 1994). Comparative developments indicate, then, that other western economies are devising new ways of financing care, but access for older people to benefits depends on the country's ideological perspectives on social policy, on their social class, ethnicity or gender, and also on their region.

Conclusion

To conclude, demographic and family structural changes mean that the older old are becoming the largest group subject to community care policies, yet reliant upon communities less equipped to care for them. It is clear, however, that many of the problems experienced are not necessarily due to the psychological processes of ageing, but to the precise wielding of institutional economic, political and social power which, harnessed to an ideology of ageism, has rendered especially elderly women vulnerable to discrimination and abuse. Social-class disadvantages too are replicated, rather than compensated for, by social policy and community care strategies. Elderly people become a football in the tussle over lines of responsibility between health and social care services. Whereas the benefits of changes in primary health are rather mixed for this user group, services for black elders seem to have scarcely changed. Social services are not able to meet the growing demand for community care from elderly people, despite the role of voluntary organisations where goals and structures are changing rapidly. Particular organisational restructurings of community care delivery and the switch from residential care to domiciliary support do not invariably enhance user group access. As ever, the central problem for the majority of elderly people is that community care policies do not serve to counteract the condition of poverty produced by class, ethnic and gender differentials in early incomes and later pensions. Care by the community is hazardous in the absence of financial security. Economies comparable to Britain are grappling with the seminal community care policy debate: Who now pays for long-term care? This is a question which no modern government has had to immediately confront until the twilight years of the current century. In the following chapter we examine specific and common issues facing disabled people in their use of community services.

Further reading

TINKER, A. (1997) *Elderly People in Modern Society*, 4th edn, London: Macmillan. The most comprehensive survey of the issues.

TESTER, S. (1996) *Community Care For Older People: A comparative perspective*, London: Macmillan. An impressive synthesis of finance, accommodation, health and social care issues in America, Western Europe and Britain.

ARBER, S. and GINN, J. (eds) (1995) *Connecting Gender and Ageing: A sociological approach*, Buckingham: Open University Press. A series of essays relating ageing and ageism to sexism and social support networks.

BLAKEMORE, K. and BONEHAM, M. (1994) *Age, Race And Ethnicity: A comparative approach*, Buckingham: Open University Press. A study of ageing and the welfare implications among Britain's black and Asian people. Comparisons with North America, Europe and Australia.

WALKER, A. and MALTBY, T. (1997) *Ageing Europe*, Buckingham: Open University Press

6

PEOPLE WITH DISABILITIES AND COMMUNITY CARE

Introduction

Analysis of community care and issues for people with disabilities necessitates discussion of how we define the group and the impact of traditional public perceptions. This area of community care is deeply marked by the ideological social construction of identity, and the related underprovision of services for people with disabilities. But the history of marginalisation has in its turn produced a distinctive collective response – some argue indeed a new social movement (Oliver, 1996) – which has placed the issue of civil rights and self-organisation firmly at the forefront of community care legislation.

This chapter examines the contested definitions of disability and the extent of disablement in British society, assesses the significance of particular trends and attitudes in relation to disability, and identifies the specific barriers faced by people with a physical impairment such as problems of access and quality of social care provision. It then proceeds to identify particular barriers facing people with learning disabilities, and to evaluate key strategies adopted in health and social care which have either empowered or disempowered; the issue of independent living and the extent to which community care policy may run counter to the very objectives of independent living; and the role of housing policies. The centrality of civil and social rights for people with disabilities is considered in the context of changing legislation and the growth of organised dissent. Finally, the chapter compares international policy experiences.

Definition

Defining disability is important, given the lack of public awareness of exactly who is disabled. Definitions by official bodies such as the World Health Organisation (WHO) and the Office Population Censuses and Surveys (OPCS) have been overly driven by the medical model of disability and fail to recognise wider aspects of disability, or they imply divergences from 'normality' which are culturally relative (Oliver, 1990). A broadening of the definition to embrace the way people are treated in society has led to the distinction between the possession of an impairment which is the functional limitation within the individual caused by physical, mental or sensory impairment, and disability which is the loss or limitation of opportunities to take part in the normal life of the community on a par with others due to physical and social barriers. Following these distinctions, Barnes (1994) and Oliver (1990) refer to 'disabled people' as 'all those with impairment, regardless of cause, who experience disability as social restriction . . . whether those restrictions occur as a consequence of inaccessible built environments, the inability of the general population to use sign language, the lack of reading material in braille or hostile attitudes to people with non-visible disabilities' (Barnes, 1994, pp. 2–3).

People suffering from mental impairment are also included in the definition of disability. To quote: 'A learning disability is an impairment of intellectual functions, which occurs before adulthood and results in significant disabilities in day to day life' (W. Midlands Regional Health Authority, 1993, p. 60, cited in Ford, 1996). The extent of their disability ranges from mild, where the person is completely independent in self-care but possesses only basic reading and writing skills, to persons with a profound learning disability possessing no self-care skills and highly limited communication abilities (Ford, 1996; Race, 1995).

The scale of disablement

A major OPCS survey of the 1980s found that more than 6 million adults in Britain suffer from one or more disability, while more than 2.5 million suffer from severe disabilities. Women are more likely than men to be disabled, while disabilities become increasingly prevalent with ageing (Brown and Payne, 1994). There are

3.7 million physically disabled women in Britain, as against 2.5 million men. Such disparities continue into old age (Lonsdale, 1990, p. 25). Estimates of the scale of learning disabilities suggest 16.5–20.5 per 1,000 with mild moderate learning disabilities, and 20.5 per 1,000 for people with severe disabilities (Ford, 1996, p. 58). Critics argue, however, that official surveys systematically under-estimate the predominance of disability by excluding those whose day-to-day activities are unhampered because of medication (Cooper and Vernon, 1996). The drawback with this particular position, however, is that the definition of disability may become so wide as to be rendered meaningless.

Issues of disablism and discrimination

Traditionally, disabled people have been 'othered' in a variety of ways, relating to how they are treated by professionals, and the models utilised to define 'disability'; the traditional institutional-isation and social segregation of disabled persons; the particular modes of discrimination; the overt prejudice encountered and the oppression experienced; and the overall ideological impact of images of disability communicated by particular media.

The medical model of disability

Although awareness and characterisation of the causes of 'disability' have expanded in the more recent period, to encompass social factors, the medical model has tended to dominate among professionals. This model views disability as a tragic event that strikes someone who 'suffers' from an impairment, thus needing medical attention which must focus on the particular impaired part of the body. Such an approach pronounces upon entitlements to state assistance, a socially controlling and legitimising function (Lonsdale, 1990). The medicalisation of disability, it is argued, is ideological in its partial and limiting perspective of the disabled person as an individual, by which the latter is turned into a victim of personal tragedy (Oliver, 1990, 1996). Measurement of the outcomes of social care and com-munity care effectiveness tends to be dominated by the medical model; thus it does not address community care objectives and conflicts with user empowerment aims (Nocon and Qureshi, 1996).

Institutionalisation and discrimination

The disabling of people must be viewed in social terms. The behaviour of social welfare institutions, and the controlling function of welfare agencies, represents institutional discrimination which serves to systematically disadvantage disabled persons, compounding the specific discrimination in various areas of human 'opportunity' (Barnes, 1994, p. 3; Goffman, 1961; Morris, 1991). Disabled people are discriminated against in labour markets, experience high levels of unemployment and many live in a state of poverty (Abberley, 1993). Yet the connections between poverty and disability are evident: 20 per cent of the world's disabled population (100 million) are disabled from malnutrition (Oliver, 1996, p. 114), although the specific conditions in western capitalist nations are certainly not comparable with those in, for example, African countries. People with disabilities face discrimination in obtaining ease of physical access and from government methods of assessment (George, 1995a). For instance, the underestimation of real need by the OPCS survey resulted in income reduction for more than one million disabled people in the 1980s (Barnes, 1994, pp. 101–2).

Prejudice and oppression

Disabled people face overt personal prejudice from non-disabled people which is reinforced by institutional policies, cultural stereotypes and labels which serve to negatively affect self-identity (Williams, 1989; Morrison and Finklestein, 1993; Davis, 1995; Harrison, T., 1995; Oliver, 1996). This prejudice is founded on such assumptions that people with disabilities feel ashamed and inadequate, they only want to emulate non-disabled people, and have no right to an able-bodied partner (Morris, 1991). Smith and Brown (1989) note a sense of parallel devaluation between the oppression and discrimination of women and that experienced by mentally impaired persons. But processes of devaluation often do cut across gender, race, class and disability. Lois Keith's experiences as a disabled woman (1996) suggest that the bulk of everyday energy is expended in deflecting the public's responses to disabled women and their stigmatising effect upon one's sense of self. Black and minority ethnic women feel the weight of multiple, total oppression as female, disabled and black (Cooper and Vernon,

1996). Despite these multiple obstacles, information on this group and its specific needs is lacking; social services departments appear unable to understand the women's experiences of racism as well as discrimination because of their disability (Francis, 1996a). In sum, institutionalised discrimination strengthens the prejudice of disablism while personal prejudice devalues the disabled person's self-esteem, intensifying the oppression of gender and racial discrimination. How this affects specific policies is now discussed.

Physical impairment, mobility and community care

Compared with other user groups, policies for people with physical impairments come well down on the community care services' priority list, are often lumped together with policies for older people and have rarely been the subject of research into their difficulties (Nocon and Qureshi, 1996). Their services receive low priority with respect to the funding of health and social care support. Most of the financial resources are spent on professionals' salaries and the more traditional facilities (Barnes, 1994). Professionals still dominate service delivery with the new community care legislation of the 1990s. The Conservative Government refused to allow people with disabilities to buy their own services in the welfare markets in spite of continued lobbying. Although government community care strategies are accompanied by statements on user empowerment and publication of Citizens' and Patients' Charters, they rarely make reference to disability or disabled citizens' rights. It is unclear whether the new care management mode of service delivery is capable of dealing with wider structural and ideological problems of disablement. Evidence indicates that real user involvement by physically disabled persons in service planning and delivery is weak (Oliver, 1996, and see also Chapter 4 of this book).

Success in community care delivery, in common with policies relating to other user groups largely depends on the effectiveness of allied policies. Solutions to problems of mobility and easy access to transport thoroughfares, buildings and the like are crucial for people with physical impairments. Yet the physical environment (transport, housing and the design of buildings) scarcely caters for the disabled person's needs. Public transport has remained

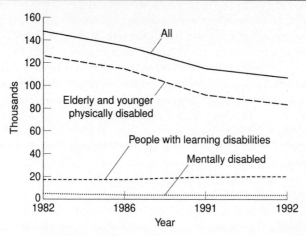

Figure 6.1 Elderly and disabled residents supported by local authorities: England. (Source: *Social Trends*, 1994.)

highly inaccessible to date, at least in Britain. Few houses are purpose-built or modified for use by physically impaired people. Many daily tasks are prohibited by a largely inaccessible built environment (Lonsdale, 1990; Barnes, 1994). A number of local authorities are involved in special accommodation schemes, but public spending cutbacks and the emphasis on owner-occupied housing serve as additional barriers (Brown and Payne, 1994).

Financial difficulties, policy and poverty

Many disabled people are in financial difficulty; social security is their prime form of provision. Possession of an impairment in itself incurs additional financial disadvantages, but the very low levels of income mean that the majority of disabled people and their families cannot meet these costs (Oliver, 1988; Barnes, 1994). As many as 47 per cent of disabled adults in Britain in the 1980s were living in poverty, according to the OPCS survey. A Family Resources Survey of the 1990s (cited in Oppenheim and Harker, 1996, p. 58) revealed that 64 per cent of households containing a sick or disabled person received no income from employment, and 27 per cent relied completely on benefits. People with disabilities face poverty because of inadequate social security benefits (Cooper and Vernon, 1996). Many, especially those with a mild impairment, have lost income since the 1988 social security reforms. Disability allowances and benefits remain insufficient for those with severe disabilities.

Again, a new 'incapacity benefit' introduced in 1995 led to lost benefits for an estimated 220,000 persons (George, 1995b; Oppenheim and Harker, 1996, p. 60). Removal of income support, under the new system of care managers, is one less direct financial entitlement to cover residential care or housework. Withdrawal of the Independent Living Fund led to similar repercussions; although flawed, it nevertheless did give disabled users direct control over their personal and support services. Now people with physical disabilities become trapped in a downward spiral of debt and illness (Grant, 1995). Social policy has evidently failed to compensate for physical and financial difficulties encountered by people with physical impairment. As we shall see, people with learning difficulties face particular institutional hurdles and a parochial social discourse.

People with learning disabilities

Society's treatment of people with learning difficulties, as we have seen in Chapter 2, has a murky history. Yet attitudes and policies have certainly changed in recent decades. Labels of 'degenerate' were attached to people with mental disabilities well into the twentieth century, 'justifying' the findings of eugenics and later Nazi social policy (Ryan and Thomas, 1987). However one detects a shift in attitudes in the increase of community services, accompanied by the development of egalitarian, integrationist and normalisation concepts intended to recreate conditions for people with learning difficulties and coinciding as closely as possible with the conditions of everyday life in the society as a whole.

Normalisation theory originated with Bank-Mikkelsen (Denmark) and Nirje (Sweden) and was refined and developed in parallel in North America by Wolfensberger, who produced a detailed technique for implementing services which enhance the value of people with learning difficulties (Emerson, 1992). Over the past twenty-five years, the trend has been against institutionalisation, and for care in the community. Changes, however, are not as comprehensive as many commentators believe. There is still the matter of how 'normalcy', which comes to view the disabled person as 'problem', is constructed in the first place (Davis, 1995). Even eugenics, argues Davis, remains on the social agenda in the guise of the new genetics in medicine (Davis, 1995) and the continuation of discrimination based upon disability in the USA, led by the Eugenics Movement (Pfeiffer, 1994).

All-Wales Strategy and community mental handicap teams

In 1983, the All-Wales Strategy, committed to Wolfensberger's normalisation ideas and supported by substantial funding for at least a decade, set up Community Mental Handicap Teams. This development represented a major breakthrough in thinking about services for people with learning difficulties (McGrath and Humphreys, 1990; Felce *et al.*, 1995; Renshaw, 1995). However, commitments seem to have waned in the 1990s: '[with] the loss of a distinctive learning difficulty policy under the umbrella of community care and the inevitable pull of competing concerns, the political shelf-life of the All-Wales Strategy is running out' (Felce *et al.*, 1995, p. 22). Enough funding has fallen away during the strategy's second phase to evoke fears that the gains of the early successful resettlement policy in meeting a diversity of individual needs are now being reversed for one of the most neglected groups in history. More generally, the period of the late 1990s is one of massive underfunding for community care services for people with learning difficulties. Major surveys by Lady Wagner and by the Association of Directors of Social Services in 1996 forecast shortfalls of £53 million in financial support to people with learning difficulties by the new millennium. The closure of long-stay hospitals leaves local authority social services in a tenuous position for assisting people with a complex set of needs within the community. Hence, their sustained refusal to fund new projects, and the reluctance to consider direct payment schemes (Valios, 1996).

Independent living, people with disabilities and community care

The notion of independent living, as presented by the independent living movement, extends across the range of human civil rights. Its philosophy is founded upon four basic assumptions: all human life is of value; all people, regardless of impairment, are capable of choosing; all people disabled by the reactions of society to physical, intellectual and sensory impairment and to emotional distress have the right to assert control over their lives; and people with disabilities have the right to participate fully in society (Morris, 1993). But, argues Morris, community care does not necessarily imply that a disabled person controls the support they need simply because it is not institutionalised. The use of friends or relatives as unpaid carers makes it impossible for the disabled person to participate – an 'enforced dependency'. Although community care policies may open up possibilities, they can also close them down. The care manager's decision-making power in the assessment process and in purchasing services for the user, plus government opposition to direct payments for disabled users, contradict principles of autonomy and participation. Morris (1993) and Morris and Keith (1995) have criticised the proponents of feminist research and the organised carer groups for silencing the voice of older disabled people by assuming the need for care, and indeed for colluding in the 'enforced dependency' strategy of community care. This position is vigorously denied by Aldridge and Becker (1996) who argue that people with disabilities and their young carers respectively remain subject to disabling barriers.

Independence and housing people with disabilities

Adequate and appropriate housing is basic on any measure of independent living. Yet the 'Living Options' Project, an important research investigation into housing and support services for people with severe physical disabilities, found that housing and support services were erratic and scarcely coordinated in the 1980s (Fiedler, 1991; Rostron, 1995). Only a fraction of Britain's general housing stock is accessible – an estimated 80,000 dwellings (Rowe, 1990). 'Special needs' housing for disabled people is often located on mainstream housing estates, divorced from the person's own support network of family and friends.

Care in the Community laid stress on the renovation grants system for the development of its community care strategy. Under the Local Government and Housing Act 1989, renovation grants were mandatory for bringing a property up to standard; under the same Act, disabled facilities grants became available and were made mandatory for providing essential access into and around the dwelling. But the grant is liable to income and capital criteria, a procedure that tends to drain clients of income which they expect to cover other living costs. Again, extensive delays in the receipt of the disabled facilities grant remain a recurrent problem in various parts of the country. Improvement grants for needs identified by community care policies have been considerably restricted due to cutbacks in government finance to local authorities (Lund, 1996).

People with learning disabilities have specific needs, and they require additional space in mainstream housing. Where they do live 'independently', much support is needed; occupants experience harrowing difficulties in running a house and organising repairs. It is crucial that their housing is located close to their social support system, but housing department allocation procedures, based on the points system, rarely embrace such factors. Nor do these departments usually possess the expertise for handling these issues effectively (Clapham *et al.*, 1990).

None of the 181 clauses in the 1996 Housing Act mentions 'special needs', or people with learning difficulties. On the other hand, the newly designated status of registered social landlords entitles them to the new social housing grant. A MENCAP official suggests that such a proposal could be used by voluntary organisations for making provision without needing to work alongside housing associations. In the meantime, 'disabled people's . . . housing rights are still not being genuinely acknowledged and continue to be masked by cash-limited assessments of care needs' (McCabe, 1996, p. 27). A major inquiry (Wagner *et al.*, 1996) reinforces this verdict on the government's silence on housing and the continuing public misconceptions regarding people with learning difficulties, perceived as odd or dangerous (White, 1996).

The independent living movement's demands for autonomy and participation, then, treat feminist perspectives and carers as contrary to such principles, although the polarity of interests is by no means apparent. What is clear is that debates over community care provision for people with disabilities raise more fundamental issues around which disability groups have mobilised.

Disability, civil rights and collective organisation

Emergent legislation over the past twenty-five years has focused on the needs and services for disabled people. However, the failure of the legislation to enhance disabled persons' rights has met with growing criticism from the disability movement. Legislation from the 1970s, notably the Chronically Sick and Disabled Persons Act 1973 (see Chapter 2) imposed duties on local authorities to produce data, while the Disabled Person (Services, Consultation and Representation) Act 1986 offered certain rights of representation and assessment to disabled persons. But the disability pressure groups found the implementation of the legislation disappointing. The thrust of the 1973 Act was not supposed to deal with socially created disability but with individuals and their presumed welfare needs; in this respect it had failed to challenge the dependency relationships (Davis, 1996).

Community care legislation and disability rights

The NHS and Community Care Act also proved as constricting in its denial of rights and in its failure to cut the dependency connection with family (Parker, 1993). 'It gives disabled people no rights', states Davis (1996, p. 127), 'and indeed has supplanted what limited rights to representation and assessment for services could have been available to us, had the government chosen to implement the relevant sections of the 1986 . . . Act.'

The very scale of the contracting out of community care services to independent private and voluntary sectors has exerted a huge impact on disabled people, ideologically undermining the legitimacy of rights, and accelerating the collapse of the welfare citizenship tradition of mid-twentieth-century Britain (Lister, 1996). Furthermore, service users' views are not receiving proper representation within the community care planning process; consultation procedures are most likely to exclude older disabled people, people with learning disabilities, people with sensory impairments and disabled people from minority ethnic groups (Bewley and Glendinning, 1994). A 1994 *Scope* survey of 2,900 disabled people and carers supported the idea that care in the community was not delivering user-controlled services (Lamb and Layzell, 1995, cited in George, 1995c).

Citizenship and disability rights

As suggested above, we may equate the continuation of discrimination in service delivery and lack of disabled users' involvement to a denial of meaningful citizenship. A number of critics argue that the individualised focus of legislation and the binding of disabled people to the welfare state constitute the disempowerment of disabled people and thus the negation of citizenship (Barton, 1993; Gooding, 1994; Walmsley, 1993; Barnes, 1994; Oliver, 1990, 1996). Community care and welfare benefits legislation emphasises 'responsibility' while minimising the significance of 'rights'; the state's role is reduced as individual responsibility is increased (Cooper and Vernon, 1996). Hence, the state's formal pronouncement on citizenship in the form of the Citizens' Charter scarcely mentions disability or disabled persons' citizenship. Care or case management may well be enhancing services for a few individuals, but it seems inadequate for solving deeper structural and ideological problems rooted in 'the disabling welfare environment' (Oliver, 1996; Walmsley, 1993; Welch, 1996).

Civil rights and the disability movement

In response to discrimination and the denial of citizenship, a Disabled Persons' Movement based on the principle of collective empowerment has developed, campaigning for the recognition of full civil rights and the introduction of anti-discrimination legislation (Lonsdale, 1990; Barnes, 1992, 1994; Oliver, 1990, 1996; Oliver and Barnes, 1993; Morris, 1993; Leach, 1996). Davis (1993) and Oliver (1996) interpret the disability rights campaign as a new social movement, which offers disabled people a political voice they have never previously possessed. On the other hand, Shakespeare (1993) treats the movement's struggles, in common with those of black people and women, as mainly to do with resource allocation rather than a reversal of values. However, organisations in the movement have been vastly underfunded and simultaneously opposed by the established voluntary organisations formerly in control of disability and in receipt of far greater funding than the self-controlled groups (Oliver, 1996). Key organisations include the British Council of Organisations of Disabled People (BCODP), set up in 1981 and representing more than seventy-five organisations of disabled people and 200,000 disabled individuals by the 1990s, and the Independent Living Movement (ILM). The shared philosophy is that disabled people will control their own organisations, but their success in forcing local authorities to accept full consultation and participation has been limited. For example, while improvements were made in the Manchester and Derby areas, the financial cutbacks of the later 1990s eliminated many of those gains (Leach, 1996).

The ILM stresses the concept of independence for all categories of disabled persons, in the sense of having control over the personal assistance needed for pursuing daily living: the antithesis of the need for care controlled by others. The movement's major activity has been to lobby against the individualistic nature of the Disability Discrimination Act 1996. Announced as the most path-breaking anti-discriminatory legislation since the 1970s and welcomed as such by the large disability charities, the Act was opposed by the disability rights movement, given the various 'let-out' clauses for employers and service providers, and the Conservative Government's refusal to set up a disability rights commission for proper monitoring of the legislation – a denial of full civil rights. The government's preferred alternative, the National Disability Council, possessed no enforcement powers. Lack of priority for good transport access for disabled people creates persistent predicaments in community care, uncovering once more official-dom's negation of a social model of disability (Chadwick, 1996; Brindle, 1996a; Braybon, 1996).

In sum, marginalisation under community care should be viewed in the wider ambit of the disability movement's focus on denial of citizenship and civil rights. This mobilisation needs to be placed in its international context.

Comparative policies for disabled persons

Policy and practice issues elsewhere are generally similar, although differences in the range of services provided exist from state to state. There is a perhaps surprising similarity in services for disabled people in Western Europe. One may detect common trends towards 'deinstitutionalisation', living in the community and the decentralisation of services. At the same time, the problems of integrated provision of services for disabled people mirror those in Britain. Italy's state provision is uneven as between the various categories of disabled people. More resources in the Netherlands, as in Britain, are being channelled into domiciliary care and away from the established model of residential care on a vast scale. During the late 1980s, Denmark devolved state responsibilities down to its 275 local authorities, many of whom, in turn, contract out to the private or voluntary sector (Wilson, 1996). Responsibility for community services for people with learning disabilities was devolved to local government after 1991 (Sandvin, 1994).

Disability benefits and financial difficulties

Although all Western European nations distribute cash benefits to disabled persons, a wide spectrum of benefits models is in operation. Countries such as France, Germany and Denmark advance care allowances directly to people with disabilities for independent purchase of domestic support services, whereas social services exert direct control in other parts of Europe, including Britain under the 1990 community care legislation (Wilson, 1996).

Disability benefits, relative to other comparable benefits, grew substantially in a number of countries through the 1970s, but then fell victim to drastic attempts at slowing down the growth. This was the case in economies as diverse as those of Australia, Sweden, Netherlands, USA and Britain. Hence, during a period of marked assertion of disabled persons' rights, people with disabilities became susceptible to long-term dependency on disability benefits. Australia, Sweden and Britain are looking more to integrate disabled people into the labour market, as a strategy for reducing the social security bill in this direction (Lonsdale and Seddon, 1994). In Britain's case, such a strategy (including the disability benefit cutbacks) has produced one of the fiercest controversies for the Blair Government (*Guardian*, 23 December 1997).

Housing and independent living

A variety of housing projects operate in European countries, many supported by the European Commission. These include fully adapted urban apartment complexes for people with severe physical disabilities in France and Belgium (the latter organised by its

National Association for the Housing of Disabled People). A scheme run by the Netherlands' National Housing Council renovates and builds dwellings which are readily adaptable in case of future disability. Denmark operates a scheme which enables disabled people to employ their own assistants for an agreed number of hours, a system which requires considerable funding (Daunt, 1991).

With respect to people with learning disabilities Italy has operated a system for handling the impacts of deinstitutionalisation from the 1970s (Wilson, 1996). Individualised funding and service brokerage schemes, for empowering and enabling independence of the individual with learning disabilities in the community were pioneered in British Columbia, Canada, through the Community Living Society (CLS). The 'community options' idea of service brokerage has spread across Europe and North America, but in many instances the schemes are operated by agencies which control the services and the funding allocations, creating a conflict of interests far removed from client empowerment (Salisbury, n.d.; Hardeman, n.d.).

The European Union

What of the role played by European government at the strategic level? The European Union spends some £56 billion per annum on programmes targeted at disabled people. The European Community Charter of the Fundamental Social Rights of Workers, 1989, recognises the need for special measures for disabled people, including assessment, transport and housing (Wilson, 1996). HELIOS has embraced 676 disability organisations, funding schemes for independent living, rehabilitation, employment, education and training. Once again, the main problem is the lack of resourcing, plus the absence of representation for disabled people. HANDYNET is a major scheme concerned with information dissemination, while HORIZON specialises in support of innovative employment projects (Daunt, 1991; Means and Smith, 1994; Hantrais, 1995; Wilson, 1996). A 1993 European Community social policy Green Paper, vociferously criticised by the Disabled Persons International (DOI), made few references to disabled people. The 1994 White Paper on European Social Policy targets the integration of disabled people and the elimination of discrimination.

Disability rights and user involvement

Wilson (1996) observes that current European policy on social integration and rehabilitation is founded on the individually based medical model of disability. Thus it fails comprehensively to counter discriminatory practice and is open to the same critiques and dissent from the disabled persons' movement campaigning for the recognition of rights. With the exception of the Scandinavian countries, user involvement is no more a reality in Europe than in Britain. European national governments seem to respond to users' needs in ad hoc fashion under the community care umbrella. On the other hand, Australia's anti-discrimination legislation (Disability Discrimination Act 1993), although not comprehensive, does offer basic rights for disabled people. Canada was the first nation to openly incorporate disability into its constitution through the Charter of Rights and Freedoms, 1982; this Charter, however applies in the public domain but not to issues of private discrimination (Cooper and Vernon, 1996). Scandinavian and American experience illustrates how legislation and litigation has managed to build a solid framework of rights for people with learning disabilities (Tyne, 1982). The key legislation in the USA, the Americans with Disabilities Act (ADA) 1990 constitutes a landmark for American civil rights. Such legislation has placed these nations in a far better light than that of most European states (Davis, 1993; Doyle, 1995; Cooper and Vernon, 1996; Oliver, 1996; Wilson, 1996).

Any such advances, however, have followed mass mobilisation and action by disabled people (Oliver, 1996). The fact of rights legislation or formal state programmes does not automatically imply that the rights are being met, necessitating continued self-controlled mass organisation in pursuit of full citizen rights. The Disabled Persons International represents more than 70 national groupings, and has tended to retreat from strategies dominated by the professional bodies. It advocates the adoption of the social model, and the incorporation of disability into the European Convention for the Protection of Human Rights and the Maastricht Treaty; the issuance of directives by the European Union supporting equality of opportunity and the provision of information; and the availability of legislation on human rights and anti-discrimination by European Union member states (DPI, 1994, cited in Wilson, 1996; Davis, 1993; Oliver, 1996). The European Network on Independent Living (ENIL), formed in 1989, has evolved gradually across the continent. But the movement's gains are constantly eroded by governmental cutbacks in funding, adding to the vulnerability of people with disabilities against the growing domination of market competition for resources, and the recurrence of disablism.

Conclusion

In conclusion, disability is more than a medical condition: it is a socially constructed situation which poses many problems for the user, and is experienced on a mass scale. Yet it is the medical model which seems to predominate, succouring medical professional power while hindering the empowerment of users, who must not only live with their impairment but also encounter grave financial difficulties, personal prejudice and related oppression. Furthermore, they face many physical barriers to mobility, not least housing and transport, which social policy as a whole has inadequately dealt with. Although formal policies have discouraged the marginalisation of people with learning difficulties, the latter are still subject to public hostility. Provision for their care remains underfunded in the 1990s. Pressures from the independent living movement underscore the significance of direct financial assistance for enabling the user to *avoid* care, and the crucial nature of specified housing provision which official housing policy has failed to recognise. Disability groups are intrinsically involved in pressuring for total civil rights and full citizenship by dint of their antipathy to the medical model and their advocacy of the social model. Their failure to substantially affect legislation is offset by an impressive raising of consciousness around the issue. Where Britain until recently resisted direct payments, some Western European nations have proved more progressive and also boast a wider range of targeted housing schemes. Resistance to user engagement in decision making may well be widespread, but Britain's legislation in comparison with that of USA, Canada or Australia, is reluctant to openly recognise citizen rights for people with disabilities. Overall, disability groups are refusing to be simply integrated into reluctant consultation procedures within the community care legislation, but are striving for citizenship rights, and spotlighting the chasm which exists between policy statements and outcomes. In the following chapter we analyse key issues for mental health service users, but especially the intricate relationships between mental illness and lack of housing.

Further reading

OLIVER, M. (1996) *Understanding Disability*, London: Macmillan. More essays by a prolific and committed specialist, concerned with disability and citizenship and the politics of new social movements.

MORRIS, J. (ed.) (1996) *Encounters with Strangers: Feminism and disability*, London: Women's Press. Critiques of the disabled people's movement from a disabled feminist perspective.

WRIGHT, K., HAYCOX, A. and LEEDHAM, I. (1994) *Evaluating Community Care: Services for people with learning difficulties*, Buckingham: Open University Press. Discusses methods of policy and financial evaluation and their application in community care.

COOPER, J. and VERNON, S. (1996) *Disability and the Law*, London: Jessica Kingsley. A useful reference.

7

MENTAL HEALTH, HOMELESSNESS AND HOUSING POLICIES

Introduction

Lack of a coordinated strategy to integrate provision for health needs with housing needs has made mental health services one of the most controversial areas of government community care policy. Deinstitutionalisation has no doubt produced a whole series of impacts on the well-being of people with mental health problems, not least homelessness. But the explanation of the latter is more complex than a one-way causal relationship, and demands closer scrutiny of public policy housing strategies, issues of service coordination and the performance of the 'new' community care. This chapter will deal with the particular relationships between mental health and homelessness, the effects of housing policies on homelessness, the series of connections between community care, the role of housing provision, and the needs of people with mental health difficulties. It will examine the impacts of mental health discharge procedures upon 'public safety' and the implications of the ensuing debate for the rights of mentally disturbed persons, evaluate the efficacy of user involvement and empowerment for mental health service users and the development of a users' movement, and finally, review comparative issues and policies.

Mental health and homelessness

An estimated 1–2 million people are homeless in the United Kingdom; the average age of homeless people is falling. Almost one-quarter of deaths among them are due to suicide (Carlisle,

1996). The nature of the relationship between homelessness and mental illness is by no means crystal clear. Many former mental patients have been discharged without accommodation provided for them in the community. But the homelessness situation itself is stressful and likely to induce depression. Again, discharged patients are prone to suffer a relapse. Studies conducted since the 1970s show that between one-third and two-thirds of residents in night shelters and hostels for homeless people suffered from a major mental disorder, schizophrenia being the most prominent. Rough sleepers on the streets experienced depression, anxiety and nervous tension. Studies conducted during the 1990s have recorded even higher levels of schizophrenia (Dawson, 1994). At the end of the century, an increasing proportion of homeless people seeking shelter exhibit a complexity of needs beyond housing; in turn, greater numbers with mental health, alcohol and drug problems require specialised provision (Fraser, 1996).

Hospital closures and discharge

Whereas the growth in the number of mentally distressed homeless persons is often attributed to the deinstitutionalisation of psychiatric hospital care and a mass discharge of patients from the hospitals (Timms, 1993), this has been happening since the 1960s and fails to explain the complete picture. One must take account of decline in hospital provision, hostels and the heightened problems for schizophrenic sufferers in negotiating their way in the community. Problems from hospital closure are compounded by inadequate numbers of acute beds, so that patients are discharged too quickly to receive the full benefit of treatment. A proportion of patients is discharged without adequate plans and preparation for living in the community, but such plans are only required for people detained under a section of the Mental Health Act 1983 (Timms, 1993; Lowry, 1991).

Direct access hostels have been more accessible and convenient, although they bear many similarities to the former psychiatric hospitals and do not offer appropriate support for homeless mental health sufferers. However, such were the poor and unhealthy conditions, that the hostels were shut down – as many as 7,000 in London between the early 1980s and 1990s (Timms, 1993, p. 102). Their replacements – secondary or tertiary referral hostels

– tend to exclude the former users of the hostel because of their stringent requirements of referral and assessment, thereby adding to the numbers of homeless people out on the streets.

Single homeless and schizophrenia

Schizophrenia sufferers are worse placed for obtaining acceptable housing and care in the community. A significant section among single homeless people, due to their disorganised thought processes, they find the protracted and complex procedures an awesome barrier for gaining access to housing. Their former hostel environment secured them a roof, but not the social stimulation needed for proper rehabilitation. For decades then, 'the result has been a dreary, demeaning *status quo* of perpetual dependence in a grim environment for the homeless person with schizophrenia' (Timms, 1993, p. 103).

Five crucial constituents of schizophrenia may contribute to homelessness: the impairment of life skills; socially unacceptable behaviour; the fluctuating course of the schizophrenic illness leading to the loss of accommodation already obtained; secondary problems such as depression or substance abuse, which may exacerbate the inability of the schizophrenic person to cope; and the sufferer's lack of insight into the nature of their disorder, encouraging a seemingly masochistic lack of cooperation.

But these are invariably affected by the social factors contributing to this group's homelessness: economic policies; housing policies and the general housing shortage; lack of familial and communal social support; inadequate support for psychiatric care from the changing community care policies; and discrimination against people with mental disorders, resulting in schizophrenia sufferers living in the worst housing accommodation (Dawson, 1994).

Single schizophrenia sufferers may well be especially vulnerable to homelessness, but the poor housing provision and absence of support from community policies worsen their plight, as explained below.

The role of housing policies and homelessness

Housing is crucial to effective community care strategy and implementation, as we have noted in earlier chapters. Conversely, housing policies have contributed to major social problems such as homelessness. Although the New Right's ideological panacea of 'market forces' as the basis of social policy has substantially affected the arenas of health and social care, the state housing sector itself has been transformed out of all recognition. A combination of overall social expenditure cutbacks, massive reductions in funding of local authority housing, and the 'Right to Buy' Housing Act 1980's inducement of sales of mass council houses and flats into private ownership. Reinforcing home ownership as a national ideology, the Act nevertheless produced a major crisis in the provision of affordable housing for groups with 'special needs' and without sufficient economic means (Forrest and Murie, 1991; Malpass, 1992; Cole and Furbey, 1994; Lund, 1996). Unhappily for community care, government funding cutbacks in local council and housing association social housing programmes represented an unprecedented 39 per cent reduction in the 1996 Budget (Weaver, 1996).

Homelessness, legislation and housing policy

This programme of housing policies, in tandem with rising unemployment, has meant the repossession of homes and the growth of 'intentional' homelessness, plus a major contraction in the size of a council house stock that could have been utilised for housing homeless persons. But how does legislation provide positive assistance? The Housing (Homeless Persons) Act 1977, incorporated into the Housing Act 1985 defines homelessness to exclude intentional homelessness and to include specific criteria. Local authorities must accord priority need to vulnerable groups, including elderly people and people suffering from a mental illness. But because of the shortage of permanent housing, these groups are invariably placed in temporary accommodation. Many local authorities deny their strict obligation by invoking the 'intentionality' clause; they tend to interpret the Housing Act 1985 in a highly capricious fashion. For example, acceptance rates varied from 3.7 per cent to almost 100 per cent of applications in 1994. The government's Housing Corporation has identified eleven categories of people who possess a 'special' housing need. Yet as we saw in Chapter 6, the Housing Act 1996, although granting enhanced powers to the Housing Corporation, neglects to mention special needs at all, while the Corporation's own rental programme was cut by 60 per cent (Lund, 1996, p. 172).

Impacts of homelessness

What of the impacts of homelessness upon health? In the 1990s, up to 70 per cent of homeless people are not registered with a GP. Homeless people are forced to use hospital accident and emergency services, which usually arrive too late and are too costly on the NHS. Ten per cent of those attending suffer from a psychiatric condition, compared with just 3 per cent who are housed. Such treatment is no substitute for proper primary care, but many GPs are reluctant to take on homeless clients (North *et al.*, 1996, cited in Rogers and Berens, 1996). Government housing policies which allow homelessness clearly run counter to the goals of effective community care policy, an issue discussed more fully below.

A major report has found that young homeless persons lacking priority status on local authority housing lists are twice as likely to suffer psychiatric disorders (Lockwood, 1996). They increasingly include young women who are extremely vulnerable to physical and sexual abuse (Douglas and Gilroy, 1994). Single parents are estimated to be eight times more likely to become homeless than other households (London Housing Research Unit, cited in Sexty, 1990; Douglas and Gilroy, 1994, p. 110).

This research, supported by findings from other similar studies, found African-Caribbean and Asian women far more vulnerable to homelessness than white women, not least because of racial discrimination. The results for these women are traumatic, leading to depression and isolation (Dhillon-Kashyop, 1994). Mental suffering by women is as likely to be caused by homelessness as it is to promote homelessness, given the traditional significance of 'home', the private sphere and the direct effects, especially on working-class females, of the built environment (Brown and Harris, 1978; Payne, 1991). Major studies in the 1980s showed unequivocally that homeless women to a greater extent than men viewed housing and domestic problems as the mainspring of mental distress and the loss of shelter as worsening their psychological insecurity (Watson and Austerberry, 1986). Homeless women on the streets face a 'double exposure'. Despite this, homeless women diagnosed as schizophrenic are less likely to have made any contact with mental health services. Appropriate accommodation is rarely aimed at homeless women suffering from severe mental distress (Allen, 1996). In such circumstances, the need for viable community care and housing policies would seem crucial.

Community care, housing provision and mental health

Housing policies may well have contributed to homelessness, but community care policies have themselves proved problematical. Both these areas of social policy undergo great difficulties in directing their strategies to the advantage of the users or potential users of their services. While the mental hospital closures do not always constitute the prime cause of increased homelessness among people with mental health problems, community care is inadequately managing the intensified rate of discharge of ex-mental patients. No new hostels were built; the old ones closed instead. The fundamental ingredient of accommodation was absent in the inner-city areas that contained high proportions of mentally ill and single people in the 1980s (Bean and Mounser, 1993).

Housing's vital part in community care was not initially recognised. Griffiths (1988) saw housing as playing only a 'bricks and mortar' role; 'Caring For People' devoted a mere four paragraphs to housing, implicitly viewing it as secondary to health and social care. Later statements and circulars, however, conceded wider responsibilities for housing, such as involvement of housing project staff in the assessment of care needs initiated by social workers (Petch, 1994). Housing schemes for this user group include independent local authority or housing association dwellings, with occasional visits from a support worker, small group-shared living schemes, and projects entailing a high degree of staff support and 24-hour nursing attention. Projects embracing support accommodation through a range of housing types and arrangements have increased in number (Means and Smith, 1994; Petch, 1994), including crisis or 'asylum' housing for people undergoing a crisis on a short- or medium-term basis (Means and Smith, 1994). Provision is nevertheless uneven and not on the same scale as for disabled people. Reports in Scotland (Spicker, 1993; Crockett and

Spicker, 1994) showed fitful service in Strathclyde through the early 1990s, no provision whatsoever in a number of districts, and a few dwellings in other districts. Housing associations in various metropolitan authorities have undertaken additional responsibilities by engaging extra support for their tenants in raising funds, but cuts in finance for special needs have hampered such initiatives.

Poor synchronisation of housing and community care

Government guidance for close cooperation between agencies is robust, as we saw in Chapters 3 and 4. But implementation has proved complex, with a multiplicity of agencies involved in shelter, health and social care. Independent working continues, regardless of initial intentions, and communication is lax (Timms, 1993; Muijen, 1996). Cooperation has not been improved by respective agencies attending to their own priorities prompted by the government's major restructuring imperatives. Many housing departments, more preoccupied with preparing for privatised delivery and new housing management systems, drew away from community care concerns in the 1980s, having worked integrally through social services' directives in the supply of 'special needs' housing during the 1970s. Government's low commitment to offer sufficient housing resources or imaginative cheap options for good community care suggests that government policy on housing completely contradicts its community care policy, which assumes total care packages involving accommodation (Rogers and Pilgrim, 1996). One detects similar contradictions in the respective agencies' underlying philosophy, which accords personal responsibility to a mentally disturbed person for their actions. Housing organisations have evicted tenants on the basis that all people are fully responsible for their actions, even in circumstances where psychiatric help is often inaccessible (Timms, 1993). If anything, the poor synchronisation of community care and housing is a cardinal reason for the disastrous outcomes in current mental health care policies.

Hospital discharge, public safety and violence

Mental health has received rather more publicity than that of other user groups in recent years because of the perceived danger posed to the 'public' when violent clients have been discharged and made homeless, sometimes leading to killings. But the policy discourse unveils a set of tensions between facilitating the human rights of people in mental distress and security rights of protection. High levels of crime exist among single homeless people; many of the men carry a number of convictions or prison records, and rates of imprisonment and arrest are prominent among mentally ill homeless persons. The latter are more likely to be imprisoned and are frequently arrested for minor offences. Up to one-half of male prisoners suffer from psychosis or organic disorder, warranting psychiatric treatment. Instead they stand at risk of homelessness on discharge from prison. Homelessness spawns violence in the search for food, money or drugs by people bereft of accommodation and necessary care (Dawson, 1994). Such violence has increased against priests on church premises in inner-city areas (Hodges, 1996). More than twenty enquiries were in preparation by the end of 1996, exposing the failures in psychiatric care, forcing government ministers to acknowledge the crisis and prioritise treatment of seriously mentally ill persons (Moore, 1996).

Violence and murder

Cases in the 1990s demonstrated the extreme consequences of ambiguous or slack community care, notably in the cases of Christopher Clunis, Kenneth Grey, Stephen Landat and Horrett Campbell. Clunis, diagnosed as a paranoid schizophrenic, stabbed a stranger, Jonathan Zito, to death in 1992, and was then committed to Rampton Special Hospital. The subsequent enquiry revealed an abnegation of Section 117 of the Mental Health Act 1983 in that no discharge plans for care in the community had been made. He was homeless for extensive periods; the psychiatric units where he was periodically admitted were underresourced and failed to keep contact with him during his other spasmodic incidents of violence. Three reports on Clunis, and on Grey and Landat, two other psychiatric patients, uncovered a number of common themes, including errors in communication, team working, community care plan implementation, the generally fragmented aspect of aftercare services for psychiatric patients still requiring support, serious underresourcing, and a disturbing lack of backup 24-hour accommodation in the community, plus the issue of 'race' and cultural stereotyping. In addition was the lapse in risk assessment (Kent, 1996). Campbell was an unemployed paranoid schizophrenic jailed for attempted murder with a machete of seven women and children in 1996, yet probation officers' recommendation for a psychiatric assessment report was rejected by magistrates only months prior to the incident (Campbell, 1996; Chaudhary, 1996).

Rights and risks

In some respects the cases above may point to the administering of stronger control measures over mentally disturbed people for public protection reasons. But decisions on risk of discharge into the community essentially impinge upon issues of the rights which belong to patients and ex-patients (Murphy, 1991). However, the climate of public hysteria surrounding this series of cases has fostered a greater defensiveness by psychiatrists and allied professionals in multidisciplinary teams. The onus now falls on patients to prove that they will not constitute a danger in the future before discharge is granted – a daunting, almost impossible task! Yet it is argued that in spite of such 'hype' publicity and 'moral panic', 'few patients with a severe mental illness reoffend and only a tiny minority kills, and more often than not they kill themselves' (Dobson, 1996). In such a climate, rights of people with mental health problems become circumscribed. The stigma of mental illness, MIND conjectures, operates when projects for hostels in the community are refused on the basis that all schizophrenics are violent killers. Acquiescence to the public mood contradicts the desirability of balancing 'the needs of the client against the rights of the public to be protected, as far as can be realistically achieved' (Austin, 1996). New legislation, the Mental Health (Patients in the Community) Act 1996, established supervised discharge orders (community care orders in Scotland) for psychiatric patients deemed to constitute a threat to themselves or to others (Whiteley, 1996).

The cases discussed reveal inadequacies in community care coordination and prolonged periods of homelessness. Clearly, whereas matters of public protection are significant, policy requires a sense of proportion in balancing public risks against the rights of mentally disturbed persons.

User empowerment and disempowerment

Under the 1990 Act, and in the wake of market-driven social policies, user involvement has become an implicit part of community care provision for people with mental health problems, as with other user groups. But what does this imply for this particular group of people? To what extent are they able to choose? How much power are they able to wield, and what of those who are severely disturbed and *must* receive support in making their voice heard?

User involvement

According to the 1990 community care legislation, mental health policy debate should incorporate user views of services, reflecting the government's managerialist ideology of consumerism and quality assurance measurement, but also the promotion of consumers' views of services by traditional pressure groups such as MIND, and the upsurge of activity among consumer organisations during the 1980s and 1990s (Davis, 1991). Social policy commentators have been less than convinced of the full acceptance of user involvement in actual decision making and a full partnership between providers and users. Alternatively, Strong (1996) cites an instance of such a partnership development during the late 1990s. The Avon Mental Health Measure scheme, involving professionals, user groups, MIND and statutory purchasers and providers, allows users and professionals to record their own assessments of needs and contribute to the formation of care package. Certainly, these are positive examples. But how much power can the groups exert?

Empowerment and the survivors' movement

The collective users' movement reflects a plurality of political positions, paralleling the rise of new social movements (see Chapter 6). The largest groups, such as Survivors Speakout and the United Kingdom Advocacy Network (UKAN) have adopted a social model, critical of the hegemonic medical model in service provision, and advocate citizenship rights (Lindow, 1995). On the other hand, other smaller groups such as Voices (the National Schizophrenic Fellowship) do not challenge the 'medicalisation' of schizophrenia, but pressurise for their own voice to be heard on service delivery (Rogers and Pilgrim, 1996). Contemporary debate within the movement, however, echoes a common theme: the reaction to users' traditional devaluation, degradation and disempowerment. It affirms the need to modify the professional–patient relationship and to facilitate empowerment, so that users may control their own lives and care services, in pursuit of the recognition of citizenship rights (including social rights) for people with mental health disorders (Rogers and Pilgrim, 1989; Barham, 1992).

Nevertheless, a disjuncture arises between mental health service users' perspectives and those of the professionals. Views held by the latter have characterised those of the former as irrational, and usually deny users' perspectives that are unsupportive of professional interests. With the growing challenge to professional dominance from managerialism and with expectations engendered by market consumerism, clinicians have only recently begun to concede the legitimacy of user views. However, one must question the extent of this 'consumerisation', given the quasi-market relations of the mixed economy and the continuing power of the NHS as 'providers' (Rogers and Pilgrim, 1996).

Advocacy

Citizen advocacy is a voluntary movement in which selected volunteers are trained by staff for representing specific individuals' interests, and providing 'legal advocacy'. Peer advocacy constitutes individual support from someone with similar experiences helping a distressed individual to obtain their wishes and view themselves in a positive light. Yet fellow professionals treat advocates suspiciously for endangering familiar power relationships.

Statutory authorities are coming to see advocacy schemes as useful in alerting them to important issues which may be missed, and for raising consciousness of users' rights; some authorities have provided financial support. But the schemes have to be independent of 'authority' professionals (Murphy, 1991). Citizen advocacy projects – for example, the Birmingham Citizen Advocacy Project – incorporate specific training programmes. Although advocacy schemes promote individuals' rights and choices, they have not really affected the functioning and planning of services, and users seem to have exercised no real influence (Murphy, 1991).

Consultation and users' groups

Rogers and colleagues (1993) have demonstrated how professionals in the psychiatric services managed to resist or ignore psychiatric patients' views in the early 1990s, either by dismissing them as 'irrational', substituting carers' views for those of patients, or by reshaping the views to suit their own professional interests. However, such resistances *are* weakening in the wake of new political forces. Nevertheless, discrimination against minority ethnic groups has led to an exclusion of black perspectives within the movement despite improved consultation procedures and growing awareness. The Psychiatric Survivors movement, articulating a philosophy of empowerment has still managed to marginalise African-Caribbean and Asian user groups, many of whom have taken alternative routes via the black voluntary sector in making their voice heard and are now involved in organised protest against insensitive services (Sassoon and Lindow, 1995).

Identification of relevant health care issues in service evaluation has relied more on professional views than on consultation with mental health service users. Social care 'quality of life' profiles for measuring adequate mental health service provision, drawn up by social services departments, have failed to address issues of independence, choice and personal control (Nocon and Qureshi, 1996). In sum, while the survivors' movements for the achievement of empowerment have raised the status of the social model and citizenship demands, and resistance to the involvement of mental health service users in consultation procedures slackens, minority ethnic voices are not heard even within the mainstream collective survivors' movement.

Comparative policies in mental health and housing

The retreat from large-scale public provision in housing, as we have observed in other welfarist areas, is not specific; elsewhere it has resulted in similar outcomes in social housing and community mental health provision.

High rates of home ownership in Britain during the 1980s were not unique. Harnessed to the ideological benchmark of market provision, the ostensible benefits brought comparable problems, as individuals became increasingly exposed to capitalist financial policies. Costs of housing grew in Western Europe, Australia and New Zealand. Similarly, the slump in house prices and general depression, for example, in Sweden, Denmark and the USA meant falling levels of private investment in housing, to the detriment of low-income groups (Doling, 1993). Low-income housing needs became progressively relegated in Western European countries into the late 1990s. Mass-scale housing problems re-emerged after the 1970s, yet few national governments support large social rented housing schemes for low-income groups (Harloe, 1994, 1995). Some 3–5 million people are estimated as homeless in the European Union member countries (Quillot, 1991, cited in Harloe, 1994). Severe homelessness exists in Sweden, where local authority social housing provision is widespread and state welfare strategies justify *exclusion* of many homeless people from social housing (Sahlin, 1995). Housing is not subject to direct intervention by the European Union, but the Commission's *Social Action Programme 1995–1997* spotlighted cooperation in housing and homelessness in an effort to deal with the widespread problem of insufficient and poor quality housing (Chapman and Murie, 1996).

United States housing policy, in common with policies for handling other economic and social problems, minimises state intervention, but like Britain the country is in a period of housing crisis. Housing provision is also of poor quality for people with mental health problems; homeless shelters lacking decent facilities or skills frequently double up as the communal facility for mentally distressed homeless people.

Homelessness, housing and mental health policy

Legislation has emerged in the United States in the 1980s to deal with the growing homelessness problem for 'special needs' groups. The McKinney Homeless Assistance Act 1987 addressed community mental health services for homeless persons. Although Congress allocated monies, these proved inadequate to meet the true scale of the problem. Health services have failed to support chronically mentally ill people made homeless. No comprehensive or integrated care system is available for this group in spite of some short-term 'outreach' programmes (such as the Homeless Chronically Mentally Ill Programme) that have made an impact in health care. Experience from general health care programmes for homeless people, though, reinforces 'the fragility of the chronically mentally ill and the difficulty in providing any semblance of care for them in the construct of a loose network of services rather than a true system of care' (Reuler, 1993). Tomlinson (1996) advocates the creation of a midpoint between complete independence and institutionalised care in the community – asylum *in* the community where intensive care is needed. But 'asylum' does not figure in official US policy owing to the antipathy of asylum to achieving 'independent' living. The Community Support Systems programme (CSS) does, however, consider the sheltered living solution (transitional sheltered living) to be an acceptable transitional arrangement towards independent living.

User empowerment and advocacy

The survivors' movement is well developed in the United States, especially in support for homeless psychiatric survivors, for example the Oakland Independent Support Centre. Survivor activities have covered permanent and emergency housing provision for shared and individual living often based upon a cooperative structure where support workers are themselves survivors.

Self-help groups involving peer advocacy have developed in the United States (Lindow, 1995). Volunteer programmes were introduced at the Houston, Texas psychiatric clinic, in San Francisco and Pennsylvania, and in Vancouver, Canada. Often the projects have encountered powerful resistance from the professionals, who resent their own exclusion from self-help groups. User-led services have been introduced in the United States. Project Release in New York, for instance, is a totally patient-directed community centre with no differentiated salaried staff (Brandon, 1995).

But the self-help movement, if not prone to mentalism, manifests an undercurrent of racism. Although offering alternatives to care in the United States, it is nevertheless a white middle-class European American social movement which has marginalised African Americans, Asians and Latinos, groups whose mental illness is more readily 'criminalised' and stigmatised, labelled a danger to the public, and hence deflected to the criminal justice system. Whereas these minority ethnic groups may hardly have featured in the 'established' self-help movement that encourages small-group participation and English speaking, these communities have formed community-wide support groups over a range of issues in many major American cities (Brooks *et al.*, 1995).

Conclusion

In conclusion, there seems little doubt that the situation of mentally distressed people exposes them to homelessness and social isolation, while homelessness *per se* increases the likelihood of mental health problems, particularly among women. Deinstitutionalisation on its own does not inevitably serve the best interests of this highly vulnerable group. Housing strategies and community care policies that operate in isolation risk a potentially disastrous scenario, especially where follow-up services are poor or simply non-existent and no stable shelter is available after a patient's discharge from hospital. Yet the general denial of rights to mental health sufferers is highly disproportionate to the frequency of criminal acts, reflecting the socially constructed poor image of this user group. The impact of community policy in increasing 'consumer empowerment' is complicated. On the one hand, the appropriateness of the social model is now widely recognised. Medical professionals, on the other hand, are very defensive in the face of advocacy and participation in consultation. In other societies, mentally distressed people also face similar difficulties of survival in the community, often without regular accommodation. Users are thus prey to homelessness, although basically white psychiatric survivor organisations are well established in North America. Mental health service users have special difficulties and thus specific needs that must be met in a fully informed and properly coordinated fashion, not least in the matching up of housing and care requirements. Major incidents have made this area of community care policy probably the most publicly controversial. In the next two chapters we examine how women and members of minority ethnic groups are experiencing community care policies.

Further reading

TOMLINSON, D. and CARRIER, J. (eds) (1996) *Asylum In The Community*, London: Routledge. Factors for consideration in providing effective community services for mentally ill people. Also international case studies.

DALY, GERALD (1996) *Homeless: Policies, strategies, and lives on the street*, London: Routledge. Studies on homeless groups, including mentally disturbed, frail elderly and people with disabilities, in Canada, USA and Britain.

MEANS, R. and SMITH, R. (1996) *Community Care, Housing and Homelessness: Issues, obstacles and innovative practice*, Bristol: Policy Press. Monograph review of research in the area, covering a range of service user groups.

LUND, B. (1996) *Housing Problems and Housing Policy*, London: Longman. Encompasses a range of policy issues, including ideology, homelessness and community care.

8
WOMEN AND COMMUNITY CARE

Introduction

Women inhabit the heart of the community care process. Their activities are based on a whole set of deeply embedded assumptions in patriarchal society with respect to 'natural' care and carers. The argument expressed in this chapter is that community care policies have been formulated on the basis that women's caring (informal care) will automatically support formal caring, but that the many stresses and strains or the economic costs are not accounted for. The chapter examines the role of women within the family network; the interrelationships between formal and informal caring for females; the role of women in the community and the considerable impacts exerted by general community and environmental changes; the significance of ageing for women faced with community care, either as carer or client; the financial hardships for women in community care and the connections with women's health; and the nature of the feminist critique of women's health.

Women, caring ideology and the family

Women in patriarchal society are invariably viewed as pivotal in caring, an activity characterised as a 'family' responsibility in the first instance. This is tied to three factors: the predominance of a biological approach to women as 'natural carers', the 'network' of females involved in caring in a family, and the prevalence of women involved through the 'life cycle' in caring.

Natural caring is a concept long adhered to in public life and socio-political literature. It is so deeply rooted as to be deemed the central feature of a female nature which becomes human nature (Cowen, 1994) and the female self-identity – the biological cause of domesticity serving to reinforce the distinction between the private and the public (Okin, 1980; Gamarnikow *et al.*, 1983; Graham, 1983; Elshtain, 1993; Dalley, 1996). This dichotomy was prominent in the nineteenth century, although events of the twentieth century, including a greater involvement of females in the workforce, contributed to its gradual breakdown. Family experts and traditional sociologists of the family have not really welcomed women's emancipation (Roberts, 1982).

Family and caring

It is undeniable that a kin network exists, developing around the person who is being cared for, and that this network usually comprises a female spouse, mother, daughter, daughter-in-law, sister and niece. The gender is female when the caring network extends to the fringes of the family, usually a female neighbour. Caring for an infirm or sick person falls to the women frequently following an initial substantial period of caring for children, compounding other domestic responsibilities of the female. The network extends beyond the family into a series of economic and social relations (Graham, 1983; Land, 1978). Clearly, women care for members of the family at different stages in the life cycle, for children, parents and then for partners (or spouses) (Ungerson, 1983b). The significance of this continuum in care, albeit broken at varying intervals, is analysed in greater detail later.

What of the male involvement in caring? Men participate in caring to a greater degree than was once generally believed (Arber *et al.*, 1988). Baldwin and Twigg (1991) suggest that the increased involvement of men may be explained largely by the specific role of the 'spouse-carer', which partly overrides the gendered division of labour in care provision. Nevertheless, the type of caring still differs, so that women undertake the 'heavy' care work, undermining notions of truly shared caring. Where men are involved in shared tasks within the kin network, it is in those tasks more concerned with ferrying and entertaining rather than with highly personal tasks. And yet again, certain areas of research do suggest that the level of state support, especially for housework, implicitly disadvantages female carers as opposed to male carers. This applies to a range of economic disadvantages to be explored below.

To summarise, notions of women as natural carers have persisted, reinforcing a private–public split which has placed a brake upon women's access to the public domain. Caring by the 'family' has constituted, in effect, a network of female carers which reproduces itself through the life cycle from parenting to caring for frail and dying elderly parents. Although it is evident that a growing number of men take part in caring within the family, usually for a spouse, inequalities remain between men and women in the burden carried and support offered from the state. But to what extent is the role of 'carer' simply an enforced external imposition? The literature suggests a complex answer.

Women as all-round carers: informal and formal care

Exploration of the ambiguities means posing the question as to why women care and examining motivations for caring which may suggest positive rather than negative connotations. Ungerson (1987) constructs a typology of caring which identifies a series of reasons for caring associated with material necessities and the context of the life cycle. She identifies the reciprocity of care as significant for women with children during the pre-school period, and the social construction of the elderly person as another infant to be cared for, caring as a legitimate alternative to paid work and caring in addition to paid work. Prevention of the 'empty nest' syndrome, caring as a legitimate alternative to paid work and prioritising health and caring in addition to paid work are relevant factors for women without children at the initiation of caring.

Yet reasons for caring also encompass love and duty. Male carers expressed their reasons in terms of the 'language of love' in the Ungerson survey. Women used the language of duty and obligation. Such differences reflect the salient distinction made by Ungerson (1983a) between caring *about* someone and caring *for* her or him. It is the latter which of necessity entails the expenditure of time on the carer's part. One may care about someone without necessarily devoting time exclusively to the experience of such emotions. Graham (1983) argues that this dichotomy between the labour and the love of caring reinforces the separation made in general discourse between the private place, the site of intimate relations with women, and the public arena of labour markets, which is about social distance (and hence incompatible with truly caring in the emotional sense). Women caring in the private sphere become defined as pursuing a 'labour of love' and thus not requiring payment. Further, the dual nature of caring – integrating labour and love – has been inaccurately treated as describing distinct territories of analysis within the social sciences. Social policy has focused on the economics of caring (that is, as labour) while research in psychology emphasises the emotional capital of caring which for women serves to define the achievement of femininity. In the process, our understanding of each facet is circumscribed. Psychological insights have undervalued the economic and political forces affecting women's consciousness. Social policy assessments, on the other hand, have prioritised the economic and devalued the symbolic significance in the construction of female identity, but these two sets of transactions mesh together for women.

Pressures to care

Women's opportunities for varying types of work are more restricted than for men's in any catalogue of women's reasons for caring. But the same kind of 'pressures' to care is experienced by female middle-class working professionals. The invocation to care rests deep within the female personality, suggests Gilligan (1982), but women may also consciously opt for the private spheres of home and family as offering greater integrity than the life of the outside public world (Elshtain, 1993). The latter interpretation portrays a female 'culture' situated on a higher moral plane than the male public domain. Lewis and Meredith's (1988) examination of how women arrive at the decision to care portrays a picture of intense emotional and material costs borne by females in caring, and concludes that even in complete breakdown, female respondents were 'glad they cared' (ibid. p. 152).

Female predominance in the caring services and community care is perhaps an obvious fact, but it is one which nevertheless highlights the interconnection of formal and informal care for women. These tasks are supplementary to females' caring tasks 'in the home' since evidence shows that very much shared care takes place in the home. Thus one may understand caring in the context of women keeping together family, economy and society. The gendered division of labour for women in the informal domestic sphere reproduces itself in the paid working context (Baldwin and Twigg, 1991). Cultural assumptions relating to the gendered division of labour have resulted in a greater acceptance of women involved in community care. Gender differentiation is thus intensified by the fact that women in community care figure strongly as both clients and carers: as nurses, health visitors, social care assistants and social workers.

Working in the independent and voluntary sectors

Women not only dominate informal care in the home and formal paid caring work, but also constitute the vast majority who work in the voluntary sector. Where payment is given on quasi-voluntary schemes, remuneration is low and the schemes are founded on the assumption that women will not only work for very little, but also develop warm relationships with the clients (Baldwin and Twigg, 1991). Paid volunteers are almost entirely female, even though general volunteering (unpaid work) does not display any obvious gender differences. Paid volunteering is closely aligned to the development of care management in the 1990s (Chapter 4). While the approach seems to promote welfare, it is also prone to deployment by policy makers as a form of financial cutback in social service provision. Baldock and Ungerson (1991) argue that the disadvantages reinscribe women's subordinate position in the society as a whole, given that the volunteer is almost inevitably female. Indeed, it is only possible to recruit people for this work at such a low wage because of women's overall position in society (such as lack of alternative work) and state policies for social security earnings and tax limits. But it must also be the case that many women *do* positively choose caring as dignified work.

To summarise, the ideological and pervasive familialism reinforced by policy assumptions that women are 'naturally' predisposed to care is a powerful explanation of why women care. But there are a variety of plausible reasons, which include material considerations, reciprocity, altruism and duty and the prioritising of health. While pressures to care build up because of declining labour market opportunities, many women consciously choose the private domain of caring despite profound hardship. Due to dominance of female labour in private caring, a greater acceptance of women working in community care exists, so that females numerically monopolise informal and formal care in statutory, independent and voluntary sectors.

Women and community

Much of the discussion in the chapter so far has focused on women's 'role' in informal caring and paid caring. But what of the changes, not least community care, wrought in the communities, and their impacts upon women both as carer and cared for ?

Women, place and environment

Community is particularly important for a large number of women negotiating the boundaries between their private, domestic world of care and home and the public arena of paid employment and struggles over welfare – in effect, the translation of the personal into the political. In one sense, this bounded space is progressive, enabling women to exert some control over their situation. However, in another sense it exerts restrictions on female choice and control, as with state community care policies. Women are more easily 'put in their place' by assuming the responsibility for offering unpaid care (Williams, 1993). Community here simply reflects the extension of the private sphere. From this angle it is unsurprising that women feel unable to turn to the community for support and for space within a society which has failed to sustain collectivist or communal values (Dalley, 1996).

A whole range of other debilitating factors such as low incomes and poor social security provision (explored later in the chapter) tend to lock women more firmly into the institutions of the household and the local neighbourhood. This is exacerbated by transport and mobility constraints. Many women have no access to a car; public transport services were drastically reduced as part of the Conservative Government's privatisation of bus and rail services. Possibilities for female carers are increasingly limited to maintain any part-time employment which demands lengthy journeys across a conurbation (Pickup, 1988). Such immobility assuredly adds to discomforts of living in the community for disabled women who regularly encounter poor physical access to social security offices and other impediments (Beuret, 1991).

Related policies will contribute to either isolating or aiding women in both rural and urban communities (Crow and Allan, 1994; Butcher *et al.*, 1993). As we saw in Chapter 1, many American and British cities have suffered profound social and communal dislocation because of economic restructuring and deindustrialisation since the 1970s. Environmental deterioration has hampered women's attempts to connect with public provision and deal with emergencies. Fear of harassment has increased. Elderly women have become more hesitant in going outdoors, so that the community 'outside' seems not to belong to them (Hanmer and Saunders, 1984).

Physical planning policies have transformed communities. The residualisation of public housing on rundown urban housing estates has notably inhibited women from going shopping, visiting the hospital and making social calls because of poor public transport. Wilson (1991, p. 152) points to the changes in the composition of family and experience of family life: 'The old, the majority of whom are women, and ethnic minorities, remain in the inner city, and are vulnerable to its crime, poverty and lack of transport.'

In sum, women stand in a rather ambivalent relationship to the community, where, on the one hand, they are more intimately involved in it than men; but, on the other hand, the environment has become too hostile for women to easily regard the community as a support for caring and a means to independence.

Women, financial hardship and community care

A key issue for women relating to community care lies in the economic insecurities experienced by those who are cared for and for those who are carers. Women carers are financially vulnerable by dint of the 'total' burden they carry in the absence of male or other family support. One may refer to an economics of work and caring, despite the fact that policies have assumed that informal female caring incurs no costs. Rimmer (1983) observes that research into caring divides costs into the direct costs of special expenses, such as diet and heating plus constant washing and cleaning, but additionally opportunity costs are forgone by not working or shortening the hours of working so as to care for a severely disabled child, a spouse or an ageing parent. Earnings are lost in both the short and long term. Chances to re-enter the labour force later are severely reduced for women effectively deskilled by a broken employment profile. Accurate prediction of future material circumstances is always tricky owing to a national economy's uncertainties, sudden unemployment and the possible effects upon different types of caring.

Poverty, females and social security

Many poverty studies have rendered women virtually invisible (Glendinning and Millar, 1991), yet more than 80 per cent of single pensioners who live on or below the poverty line are female. Household income figures obscure the poverty situation of women within families. Poverty is experienced by a majority of married women residing with a male partner, but also by unmarried women providing considerable amounts of care for an ageing dependent relative (Glendinning, 1988).

Women's road to hardship is hastened by the British pension system. Female dependence upon a spouse's pension, whether public or private, has meant meagre financial assistance for women in their later years. In other countries such as the Scandinavian economies, the state possesses a higher profile in providing pensions. New mechanisms *vis-à-vis* SERPS calculations in Britain and the reduction of the SERPS widow's pension to 50 per cent of the deceased spouse's pension as from the beginning of the twenty-first century will increase the incidence of poverty among elderly women (Ginn and Arber, 1994). Where employment is broken, occupational pensions fail to provide women with independence later in life (Ginn and Arber, 1994).

Male–female differentials for invalid care allowance

Because of the Beveridge assumptions which denied benefits for women, an Invalid Care Allowance (ICA) for carers did not materialise until 1974, mainly stemming from formal political pressure by single female carers of elderly parents for a non-means benefit entitlement. The eventual ICA excluded married women (again owing to a Beveridge assumption of wives' 'automatic duty' and 'natural caring' instincts (Groves and Finch, 1983). This was a clear case of gender-specific social policy reinforcing traditional patriarchy. Invalid Care Allowance was only granted for married women in1986, following a European Court of Justice decision.

However, the ICA seems insufficient for replacing lost earnings and falls woefully short of what is necessary for ensuring an independent income for carers (Baldwin, 1994). Furthermore, the majority of carers do not receive ICA, since the latter excludes a number of categories such as pensioners. Only one-tenth of carers exceeding more than thirty-five hours per week care were in receipt of ICA in the1980s (McLaughlin, 1991, cited in Baldwin, 1994). Female carers in fact suffer severe hardship when, for example, a mother is refused attendance allowance (Lewis and Meredith, 1988).

Policies on caring, then, have wrongly assumed no costs for female carers, yet denial of alternative earnings' compensation has culminated in severe financial hardship and dependency for female carers, in the absence of any radical operation in employment and social security policies. Special Allowance entitlements are in the minority and male carers are more likely to benefit than female carers, while difficulties are compounded by the carer's own health, discussed in the next section.

Women, health and community care

Gender plays a part in affecting the likelihood of a person needing care due to sickness, disability or general ill-health. Men enjoy better health at a number of age ranges; elderly women suffer more physical impairments and incapacities than men and undergo more severe cognitive impairment above the age of 80, and they suffer serious disadvantages in age-specific functional disability. Twice as many women as men over the age of 80 are 'severely' disabled, and hence more likely to need both informal and formal caring. Such cumulative health disadvantages are hastened by elderly women's inferior financial situation (Arber and Ginn, 1991).

The poorer health is also affected by the greater weight of household tasks for women, contributing to high rates of depression (Brown and Harris, 1978; Doyal, 1995). The demands of caring for sick and disabled adults can extract a physical and emotional toll exceeding even those for tending children, especially the emotional stress not usually present in bringing up children (Ungerson, 1987; Lewis and Meredith, 1988). This also raises the perennial question: Who cares for the carer? The answer is often 'no one' in households where women are expected to carry burdens alone and in the 'society' where government frequently abdicates responsibility (Doyal, 1995). Such women entering the early phases of old age, notably married women below retirement age caring for elderly relatives, appear most susceptible to stresses, since the caring demands are most likely to clash with competing family responsibilities, personal career and opportunities of accumulating an occupational or private pension (Arber and Ginn, 1991). Waerness (1990) refers to this group as the 'middle generation', which may find themselves in a 'stressful bridge position' between the generations, the strain compounded by the growing divorce rate among the younger generation (ibid. p. 128).

Debates on the feminist critique of caring

Much of the literature on gender and community care over the past few years has been inspired by feminist perspectives, but as the 'field' has developed, any obvious consensus has evaporated. Feminist research has mounted a powerful assault on patriarchal welfarism since the 1970s, identifying the discrete ways in which community care policies are de facto resourced by women's unpaid labour. Feminists construed gender divisions within the family as the mode whereby community care policies reinforce women's economic dependence, counteracting policy makers' claims that community care supports the social independence of care recipients. Finch (1984) openly rejects community care in favour of expanding institutional care (at odds with the deinstitutionalisation movement influenced by Goffman), on the basis that 'family' support in community care was basically care by women. These analyses clearly underpinned the case studies and empirical investigations. Dalley's (1996) reassertion of collectivist values questions the whole ideological framework of care policies and their inextricable linkage with gender marginalisation. Her essential argument is that the 'possessive individualism' assumed in social policies is a gendered concept which only fully applies to men, who view 'family' as the private retreat in their lives. Collectivist and communal alternatives for caring, she observes, have received no proper attention, yet these are always possible and indeed necessary for offering disabled and dependent people the responsibilities for making real life choices. Yet although the feminist research perspectives of Finch, Groves and others seemed to express uniformity, the critiques of their position have been largely ignored.

The critiques of feminist perspectives

In the first place, the feminist world-view does not match *all* female experience, but rather that of white, heterosexual women. Second, feminist case studies have focused on carers – the givers, as opposed to the recipients of care (Begum, 1990). Third is the position (shared with the researchers themselves) that many women with disabilities are self-caring and 'service' the other family members at the same time (Begum, 1990; Morris, 1991). Morris (1991) argues that no unequivocal choice exists between community *or* residential care, and that slight attention is paid to disabled and older persons' experiences of physical and emotional abuse, which happens irrespective of setting (that is, community and residential care). Her observation that residential care does not constitute the sole alternative to assistance at 'home' challenges the earlier feminist position, which overemphasised women as carers, thereby underating the numbers of male carers. The common assumption that men would not wish to care for a disabled partner remains a highly questionable one for Morris. Furthermore, research (Arber and Ginn, 1989) demonstrates that depending on the level of disability, the type of household is more significant than gender in determining who provides the support to elderly infirm males and females.

Again, early feminist research tended to create too sharp a dichotomy between carers and cared for, thereby missing the extent to which older and disabled women also act as carers. When articulating which of those policies should or should not be supported, even Dalley's collectivism and stress on empowering persons with disabilities with responsibility for life choices deny them a direct hearing. The capability of collectivist forms to break down male–female inequalities, however, when a community is formed for caring for people with disabilities, is suspect. Notwithstanding, Baldwin and Twigg (1991) call for greater attention to communal forms of living structured around social, cultural or religious identities, so as to facilitiate women's greater choice over caring decisions.

Comparative policies

Theoretical and empirical comparative material on the gender impacts of community care, and indeed social policy, is in short supply. This significant dimension has been clearly neglected by major comparative welfare state analyses, such as Esping-Andersen's (1990) *Three Worlds of Welfare Capitalism* which probes the effects of social security spending. In the same vein, there remains a paucity of comparative policy analysis on ethnic dimensions (Ginsburg, 1992; Tester, 1996a). And again, to what extent is familialism an international phenomenon?

'Family' and financial social policies

Familialism as an ideology underpinning social policy is not unique to the British case. But it is also transparent that a distinct 'familialist' bias in pensions and the provision of welfare services is more prevalent in Britain and continental Europe than in Scandinavian economies (Esping-Andersen, 1996). Whereas Britain's state pension policies have tended to reproduce women's financial dependence, which is detrimental to their economic security, social policies have been 'gender neutral' in Denmark (Siim, 1990). Because of their unequivocal presence in insured paid employment and eligibility for a range of employment-related benefits, including pensions and welfare entitlement, Swedish women's situation compares very favourably with that of their counterparts in Canada, USA, Britain and Germany, even though women's position within Sweden still reflects historical national assumptions regarding their dependent status (Dominelli, 1991; Ginsburg, 1992).

Women and caring

Care policies have now switched from the institution to family networks and the independent voluntary sector in many countries, even where welfare state traditions are strong, as in Scandinavian polities. Greater recognition is currently afforded to women's caring labour and to the importance of supporting carers in the home in France and Britain (Tester, 1996b). But with state expenditure cutbacks derived from tighter financial strategies, more responsibility reverts to women within the family and the wider community. Germany's patriarchal ideology is more forceful than in Britain or France. Through a series of basic laws frequently contested by the women's movement, policies of social market economy have been strictly traditionalist towards the role of women and the family. Indeed, future obstacles are anticipated in the recruitment of paid care workers in countries like Germany and the Netherlands, probably affecting women employed as cheap labour from disadvantaged economies of Eastern Europe (Tester, 1996b).

Conclusion

To conclude, in this chapter we have analysed the importance of familialist ideology in caring, women's numerical domination in informal and formal care, and the range of explanations for why women care. We have also examined the marginalisation of females from community networks and the impacts of traditional welfare policies in causing crippling financial hardship. It would be churlish to deny the power of the familialist explanation justifying female caring as natural, one which simultaneously rationalises the private (female):public (male) dichotomy in patriarchal capitalism. But it is an insufficient explanation which rules out the idea that women may consciously prioritise caring for reasons such as a genuine altruism, direct material considerations and the positive preference for authentic private relationships over inauthentic public relationships in the labour market. Restructured communities undoubtedly cause particular hardships for carers and females who are cared for. Financial adversity, however, leads to additional debilitating circumstances, such as low lifetime earnings, poor pensions and a minimal level of care allowance, comparing unfavourably with benefits for men. The relatively poor health endured by women adds to the economic difficulties. Finally, while the early feminist critiques of caring and caring policies were extremely influential, there was no single, undisputed voice but a plurality of voices. Some are the voices of carers, others are those of the cared for who seek independence from other women or from institutions, all of which foster dependency.

Further reading

UNGERSON, C. and KEMBER, M. (eds) (1997) *Women and Social Policy: A reader*, 2nd edn, London: Macmillan. Spans the policy range, including community care and European experience.

DALLEY, G. (1996) *Ideologies of Caring: Rethinking community and collectivism*, 2nd edn, London: Macmillan. Classic feminist critique of the community care model and familialist ideology. Adopts a collectivist perspective.

BUBECK, D. (1995) *Care, Gender and Justice*, Oxford: Clarendon Press. A testing but lively review of the philosophical debates.

SAINSBURY, D. (ed.) (1994) *Gendering Welfare States*, London: Sage. Investigates the impacts of welfare state policies on women and men in European economies.

9
MINORITY ETHNIC GROUPS AND COMMUNITY CARE

Introduction

Community care as between ethnic groups is far from equal. Yet Britain is a multi-ethnic society. Ethnic minorities in Britain number more than 3 million people or 5.5 per cent of the total population. Black Caribbeans form approximately 1 per cent of the total, almost 500,000 people; 2.4 per cent of the population are of Indian or Pakistani origin (approximately 1,317,000). The Chinese population (163,000) and the Bangladeshi population (157,000) each constitutes some 0.5 per cent of the total (1991 Census). Because of the statistical ambiguities, the sizable Jewish population of an estimated 308,000 does not appear in the Census as a differentiated ethnic group, but statistical estimates have been independently conducted (Haberman and Schmool, 1995). (Curiously, this issue is not identified or recognised in the Fourth PSI National Survey discussion of the 1991 Census and diversity of origins.) The matter of community care for the Jewish community has correspondingly received scant coverage in the care literature. British Jewry is concentrated in only a few areas of Britain – now mainly London, Manchester and part of the South East England coastal area, with concomitant and growing demand for community care. The Black and Asian populations are highly concentrated in the London area, Birmingham, Leicester and Bradford, whereas the Chinese community is much more dispersed.

This chapter will consider the various facets of racism and 'othering' that have affected all of these groups, racial discrimination experienced generally, and particular spheres of community

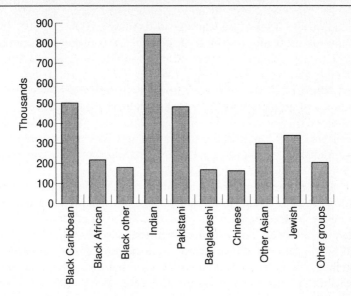

Figure 9.1   Britain's minority ethnic population. (Source: 1991 Census of Population; S. Haberman and M. Schmool, 'Estimates of the British Jewish Population 1984–88', *Journal of the Royal Statistical Society A*, 158, 547–62.)

care provision. It will explore the situation of family or informal caring in the African-Caribbean and Asian, Chinese and Jewish communities, and then focus on particular issues of voluntary sector provision in the Chinese and Jewish communities. Finally, it will make comparisons with community care and the treatment of ethnic minorities in other western economies.

Racism and 'othering'

It is difficult to survey the situation of minority ethnic groups in relation to community care and social policy without discussing the ideological pressures from racism experienced by these groups. Until the 1960s, racism was defined as a dogma: a set of beliefs usually bound up with the concept of biological hierarchy. Since that time it has come to incorporate a complete set of practices and attitudes and not just beliefs: 'in this sense racism denotes the whole complex of factors which produce racial discrimination and sometimes . . . racial disadvantage' (Cashmore, 1996, pp. 308–11). While racism is now legally unrespectable, it continues to operate de facto, perpetuated through a subtle shift away from the transparently abusive and prejudicial towards more covert institutionalised forms of discrimination. Although Britain's minority ethnic groups are very different in origin and cultural, social and religious practices, they do share the common experience of being excluded from social and political institutions, and of confronting racist attitudes, practices and racial discrimination (Solomos and Back, 1996).

As we saw in Chapter 1, 'community' is a double-edged concept, in that its very criterion of inclusiveness must imply exclusion for some, while the damage wrought to communities in a 'multi-ethnic' Britain has been far-reaching over the past decade (Husband, 1996). But of course historically the process of exclusion extends much further back. Williams (1996) identifies three modern historical moments illuminating the relationship between racial politics and the politics of community care. In the first instance lay the effects of the Aliens Act 1905 and immigration controls targeting Jews, who were given little option but to turn to self-help community care. Second was the influence of the eugenics movement in the interwar period, which promoted the pathologising and 'othering' of specific social groups, and served to shape this century's welfare policy. Third was the pathologising of black people. This has affected the postwar experience of African-Caribbeans living in Britain so much that many of the elders, it is believed, are returning to the West Indies; as such, policy makers in health and community care have tended to devote less attention to this community's requirements (Blakemore and Boneham, 1994). With respect to the Asians' overall experience, they sense a 'disinterest' projected by white British professionals. Many older people either live on their own or with sons and daughters in 'distancing' suburbs, disillusioned with their 'othered' status in Britain.

Racial discrimination

The Race Relations Act 1976, which set up a national Commission For Racial Equality (CRE), was introduced to deal with cases of alleged discrimination, but the results in terms of successful prosecutions have been disappointing and ineffective, although the dissemination of anti-discriminatory publicity and codes of practice has proved valuable (Blakemore and Drake, 1996). The NHS has demonstrated implicit resistance to its investiture of anti-racial discriminatory statutory duties. Minority ethnic groups are still greatly underrepresented in the NHS; unequal health care survives, reinforced by a history of 'race relations' policies in the health service comparing unfavourably with many large private sector companies (Law, 1996).

Racism and the process of 'othering', then, may be seen as more than dogmatic biological determinism: its discrete forms, incorporating cultural boundaries, are more opaque. Minority ethnic groups have been excluded from the broader community at different historical junctures, from the Jews in the early century to black African-Caribbeans and Asians during the postwar period, and subjected to myths of communal parochialism. Yet anti-racial discrimination legislation introduced by the state is still less than effective, not least in areas of the NHS. But how has the history of racial discrimination particularly manifested itself within community care?

Racial discrimination and community care services

As suggested above, resistance to anti-racism policies intimates an institutional antipathy from NHS professionals towards black minority patients. Viable participation of local black groups in local health policy formulation and service delivery diminished with the tightening grip of the national state in the 1990s (Law, 1996). Health services are racially discriminatory as experienced by black African-Caribbean and Asian communities, documented by a range of research studies (Ahmad, 1993). Issues of racism arise at the levels of direct racism, for example staff intolerance and racism at an organisational level, culturally inappropriate facilities and institutional racism by allocation to the worst hospitals of disproportionate numbers from black minority groups (Blakemore and Boneham, 1994).

Chapter 3 has already discussed the racist assumptions supporting practice in British mental health services. Patel (1993) detects a tacit lack of urgency for meeting black elders' needs, reflected in

181

the widespread absence of language facilities among general practitioners; she advocates special education and training of health professionals with respect to black elders' care. Black women have also suffered from inferior quality health care, rooted in historical patterns of racism and sexism (Mama, 1992).

Social services and community care

A consistent issue for minority ethnic groups is the paucity of knowledge about service availability and the underutilisation of services, especially among older and non-English speaking people (Butt and Mirza, 1996). For example, an investigation into informal care among Chinese elders discovered that the majority had received no assistance from social workers, community nurses or home helps, or benefited from meals on wheels. Services were either inaccessible or unknown to the Chinese elders, or considered inapplicable (Butt and Mirza, 1996). The current Fourth PSI Survey (Modood *et al.*, 1997) reveals a generally less frequent use of health and social services among Chinese and South Asians.

Black elders' experience is mirrored in the many impediments to regular engagement with social services. These include recurrent problems such as merely receiving 'one-off' commitments from local authorities, the latter's deployment of existing personnel instead of acquiring more relevant staff, the failure to budget for special projects, and inappropriate, mediocre meals services (Blakemore and Boneham, 1994). A study conducted in Gloucestershire found that some 40 per cent of black elders had no awareness of the county's social services. Difficulties of access to day services and their restricted choice were expressed by at least 30 per cent of the Asian elders (Social Services' Inspectorate *et al.*, 1991).

Although the 1990 legislation on the whole improved the recognition of assessment procedures, it has not led to more effective needs' assessment for minority ethnic groups, as previously noted (Chapter 4). Cultural insensitivity continues, with limited cash budgets only earmarked for these assessment procedures. Any general progress made by social services since the 1990 Act is uneven (Luthra, 1997). Eligibility criteria remain controversial, as with interpreting difficulties and the restrictive care packages for groups such as the Chinese. Consultation with minority ethnic groups is somewhat tokenist (Law, 1996; Walker and Ahmad, 1994); there is the additional failure to conscientiously apply anti-racist social work perspectives in documenting specific discriminatory practices in care management and care provision (Law, 1996). Indeed, the social work educational body CCETSW was pressured by the Conservative Government to dismantle its overt anti-racism curriculum, attacked as too 'politically correct' (CCETSW, 1995; Skellington, 1996).

Health services would seem to represent a territory of both implicit and explicit racially discriminatory practices and attitudes, with minority ethnic groups receiving inappropriate treatment, which suggests a pressing need for more health professionals from minority ethnic groups. Chinese, African-Caribbean and Asian communities experience psychological distance from the services, especially among the community elders; cultural insensitivity is typical, needs assessment procedures are cursory or inappropriate, and professional anti-racist mission statements are rarely applied to the monitoring of provision. Family care, however, provides another potential site of implicit racism.

Family care and minority ethnic groups

Generally, little is known about the informal caring in these communities, although it is believed to be similar to that among the white population. But shaky assumptions are adopted about the extended family networks for supporting elderly and disabled people (Walker and Ahmad, 1994; Atkin, 1996; Atkin and Rollings, 1996; Butt and Mirza, 1996). What is the situation among the respective minority ethnic groups?

Family care in African-Caribbean and Asian communities

Given the invisible character of informal caring, white service providers tend to assume that there is no need to offer support for minority ethnic groups. Hence, black and Asian carers figure among the least supported. The diminishing overall family size in Asian communities exacerbates the situation. As in the white population, more daughters and daughters-in-law are now in full-time employment, yet the caring tasks fall to the women. In this respect, although the financial consequences of caring are comparable, minority ethnic groups' employment prospects are poorer and greater difficulties confront their members in acquiring all their social security entitlement (Craig and Rai, 1996). Hence, the daily context is one of poverty for many black users and carers (Law, 1996).

Britain's Southern Asian 'immigrant' communities, previously in close contact with family back home, are now ostensibly undergoing radical changes akin to the status of 'autonomous' minority accorded to British Jewry, and possibly auguring the fragmentation of traditional community supports. Blakemore and Boneham (1994) posit that the feasible replacement of such support systems by more institutionalised and different models of care, as with the growth of Jewish old persons' homes, could mean a stressful period 'as family obligations and roles are renegotiated'. But American evidence suggests that 'caring and other social relationships between older and younger black people stand the test of time *better* than among whites' (ibid. p. 37).

Family care in Jewish communities

Family care is still strong in Britain's Jewish communities. While it is true that the more professionally orientated younger generations are accordingly more socially and geographically mobile than earlier generations, any decline in family care is felt to be less extensive than in other communities (Manchester Jewish Care Services). As in the society as a whole, a larger proportion of the Jewish population is elderly and growing numbers are living alone without close family on hand. This is more of a quandary in the smaller and declining communities such as Merseyside's Jewish population, located in an economically depressed region where many of the younger generation have moved out in search of employment. In response to the trends, local Jewish welfare organisations are having to expand their carers' support systems. Although the contemporary decline in family care is less pronounced in Jewish communities, larger numbers of elders without accessible family and requiring care constitute a challenge for Jewish care support services.

Family care in Chinese communities

With the increased occupational and social mobility of the younger British Chinese generations (Modood *et al.*, 1997) the Chinese extended family in Britain is diminishing in importance, particularly in the smaller Chinese communities. Members of the younger generation frequently move to the larger cities to work, leaving Chinese elders on their own, but reluctant to reside in local authority homes. Assessing the deeper ramifications of waning family care is problematical in the absence of detailed information. For instance, the current PSI National Survey (Modood *et al.*, 1997) is unable to show separate statistics for the Chinese community.

There is no common position, then, regarding family caring patterns across the minority ethnic communities. Despite the myths of 'returning' elders or of the permanent extended family, financially constrained African-Caribbeans and Asians perform caring tasks unsupported by the state. Yet again, as a consequence of new generational mobility profiles, Britain's Chinese communities are no longer able to maintain the traditional extended family network, but the future implications are difficult to gauge.

The voluntary sector: charities and mixed provision

In Chapter 4 we discussed the encouraging successful development of black voluntary organisations in the 1980s, providing a clear intimation that one ought not to view black communities as 'victims' which much 'race' literature appears to imply (Atkin, 1996). Self-help agencies – for example, the Black Health Workers and Patient Group and the African-Caribbean Voluntary Help Association – proliferated during the 1980s in response to problems of health care provision (Grimsley and Bhat, 1988). This was the case in other minority ethnic communities, interpreted as a 'turning away from the state for solutions' (Etherington, 1996, p. 10). But as we have recorded, the weakening of the black voluntary groups through the new 'contract culture' has nullifed many of the early gains in autonomy. The experience of minority ethnic groups is a differentiated one, however. Here we concentrate on the less researched Jewish community, and on key issues engaging voluntary bodies.

The Jewish community and community care

Jewish communities during this century have spawned a plethora of Jewish welfare organisations, a tendency arising out of the early marginalisation of the Jewish community which followed the waves of immigration at the turn of the century, the subsequent oppressive Aliens Act, the community's notable religious pattern and its tradition of charity (Alderman, 1992). A refocusing of Jewish welfare organisations was necessitated, however, with the development of the postwar welfare state. For example, Manchester's Jewish Social Services concentrated upon special needs for young, very old and mentally disturbed people (Williams, 1988). But until recently such charitable organisations had not been professionally administered, and exerted very little influence with local statutory authorities. With the ageing of the Jewish population, Jewish communal welfare agencies have been pressured to amalgamate and rationalise. The result in London was the formation of Jewish Care in 1990, which became the nation's biggest Jewish welfare agency offering residential and domiciliary facilities at 33 separate centres (Alderman, 1992).

In the past, Britain's Jewish community, because of its relative wealth, felt able to adopt a blanket self-help policy, but the decline in its size and the growing pressures for community care have resulted in a more pragmatic attitude and the granting of central government financial assistance (Alderman, 1992). The NHS and Community Care Act's requirements for local government to substantially engage voluntary providers has resulted in a much closer liaison between Manchester's Jewish voluntary services (serving a 35,000 population) and the region's local authorities. The last few years of community care policy witnessed a marked improvement in the professionalisation of the area's Jewish social services, including the formation of a Jewish Community Care Forum which has contributed to Greater Manchester community care plans (1993, 1995), a newly amalgamated Federation of Manchester Jewish Social Services, a higher profile of contracting for services and a growing team of qualified social workers for conducting community care assessments. As a result of the 1990 legislation, Manchester Jewish Social Services' income grew from £11,000 per annum in 1992 to £125,000 in 1995 (data obtained from the Manchester Jewish Social Services, 1996). Closer contact has encouraged greater sensitivity to religious and cultural care needs and a generally improved cultural awareness.

The scale of the statutory–independent sector interactions in Manchester nevertheless contrasts with the situation of Merseyside's much smaller Jewish community (3,500). The Merseyside Jewish Welfare Council provides support services, but does not possess the same infrastructure as its North West neighbour for supporting contracted activities. It emphasises the provision of day services for the elderly population and tends to work alongside the local authorities, but argues that the involvement of many volunteers from the community and the availability of the community's Jewish old age homes constitute a distinctive and popular service which the statutory local authorities are not able to provide.

Whereas gains have been forthcoming in the major centres, independent providers face problems, the biggest of which is common to all community and voluntary organisations: the drastic cutbacks in funding to the voluntary and independent sector by local authorities during the second half of the 1990s. This coincides with a period in which the numbers of elderly Jewish people requiring community care have multiplied. Another difficulty is that the 1990 Act's stipulation of choice is unrealistic for a Jewish provincial community of 35,000 people with only four residential and nursing care homes. Manchester's Jewish community also faces the challenge of the rapid contemporary growth of its ultra-orthodox groups, but lacking the resources of London's Jewish social services to meet the rising large-scale demand for orthodox religious community care. Finally, Jewish organisations suggest that 'cultural sensitivity' training within health authorities and social services has inadequately conveyed any deeper understanding of orthodox religious home care service and meals' requirements. This situation is not helped by the rapid turnover in hospital staff who have benefited from professional training.

In contemporary Britain, the Jewish population does not fit so neatly into the category of a racially discriminated against ethnic group, relative to African, Caribbean or Asian communities where most members are easily identifiable by colour. This, however, veils a more complicated picture. Historically, Jews have suffered from racial and religious persecution. Although the British situation does not compare with the anti-Semitism of the European continent, the phenomenon has nevertheless persisted in this country into the 1990s (Runnymede Commission on Anti-Semitism, 1994). It is therefore troubling that social work training has not really addressed anti-Semitism. Roskill (1994) proffers a variety of explanations for this oversight. Initially, many staff or student social workers have never had a Jewish client, owing to the highly proactive nature of Jewish welfare organisations. Additionally, Jews are not associated today with the victims of oppression. A number of social workers, including Jews, are ambivalent about Zionism. Yet there is still much ignorance about the facts of the Holocaust and its aftermath. Many Jews have wished to believe that the Holocaust finally obliterated anti-Semitism as a live force, and hence have felt that to raise the matter of anti-Semitism seems an irrelevance in discussions on social oppression. To quote Roskill (1994, p. 25): 'Some Jewish social workers have kept silent because we have not wished to distract anti-racism from its frequent focus on racism connected with colour.'

In sum, although statutory authorities are now paying more attention to links with Jewish communities, the traditionally low cultural sensitivity in service provision is at least partially rooted in an institutional anti-Semitism which has been accorded less recognition than racism founded on colour.

Chinese community voluntary care

Based on discussions with a small Chinese community in Gloucester-shire, it is plain that much of the community care is being conducted by a tiny, poorly supported voluntary sector organisation, comprising a Women's Guild and a men's centre: volunteers basically carry out most of the duties with respect to the administration for hospital entrance and access to social care functions, home visit services and advocacy service. An Elderly Chinese Day Centre was instituted in 1992, run by the Chinese Community Group.

But the problems experienced indicate a more general marginalisation of Britain's Chinese community. Language communication barriers mean that the first generation of immigrants stemming from the Chinese villages are not able to communicate their needs to hospitals or GPs. Constant demand for the voluntary services also reflects the older Chinese community's suspicions of state interference in domestic circumstances. It is argued that racial discrimination seems to inhabit the statutory bodies' general lack of cooperation and assistance and that cultural insensitivities persist. For instance, no local authority policy is in operation for keeping together people who have only known other members of the Chinese community. Services provided by the statutory authorities also display poor cultural awareness in the lack of proper facilities, minimal interpretation assistance and inappropriate meals services.

The Chinese community, then, personifies exclusion, certainly as it pertains to care services, because of language drawbacks among its elders, and suspicion of statutory institutions which have failed to anticipate the community's particular cultural needs.

Comparative policies

Although minority ethnic groups include some of the most disadvantaged communities in many countries, official statistics are sparse on the effectiveness of the welfare state in accommodating their needs (Ginsburg, 1992; Bryson, 1992; Hantrais, 1995). In this section we will focus on issues of discrimination relating to social support and the particular treatment of black elders.

Racial discrimination and welfare

Racial discrimination is widespread, although attempts vary to counteract its incidence. Certainly, available evidence points to underutilisation of health services by minority ethnic groups in a number of countries. In Sweden, erstwhile social democratic but currently in the midst of political ideological transformation, no equivalent exists to Britain's Commission For Racial Equality. Sweden's new ethnic minorities seem to have become a 'racialised' underclass: non-Nordic people are subject to discrimination from the nation's immigration control policies. Furthermore, the habitual eugenic attitude towards race and immigration continues, although implicit rather than overt (Ginsburg, 1993). Despite the more progressive social democratic welfarist policies, the new ethnic minorities do appear relatively more dependent upon means-tested benefits (Ginsburg, 1993).

Minority ethnic groups in Germany since the 1970s have been in receipt of certain welfare benefits, such as social assistance, reflecting state response to pressures from minority ethnic communities. Yet they remain net contributors instead of beneficiaries of the social security system. Pathologisation of 'the black family', whose economic circumstances are constructed as 'social problem' as distinct from an issue demanding urgent policy action, has a protracted history in the USA. Black people are automatically labelled as 'underclass' and as 'prone' to drop into the poverty category (Ginsburg, 1992; Weir, 1993).

Elders

One-third of elderly black people, compared with approximately one-tenth of older whites, fell below the poverty line in the USA during the 1990s. Along with females, this group bears the brunt of the Medicare insurance scheme expenses, while upper and middle classes enjoy the benefits (Tester, 1996a). As a general rule, the black elder population forms a substantially larger 'minority' than in Britain, accounting for its greater confidence. Britain's many established early migrant communities still face the prospect of a permanent lack of acceptance (Tester, 1996a), although the myth that few 'minorities' require formal care because of the 'return home' belief prevails in other societies too (Hugman, 1994).

Conclusion

In conclusion, minority ethnic groups still experience exclusion from quality public services and community care, regardless of the introduction of anti-racist legislation and the promulgation of anti-racist charters. The health services remain a site of discriminatory practice, cultural insensitivities and inappropriate treatment, alienating many minority ethnic elders. If family care does appear to be stronger than in white communities, it varies in degree as between African-Caribbean, Asian, Jewish and Chinese populations, as does the capacity of ethnically oriented voluntary organisations to support family care. The immediate relevance for statutory bodies of the Jewish community's caring structures is now greater by dint of contemporary contractual arrangements with local authorities. Language represents the major barrier for the Chinese community, which must manage the considerable challenge of ensuring adequate community care provision through inadequately resourced voluntary structures, especially in smaller centres. Finally, the British situation for minority ethnic groups is by no means unique, not least because of the minimising of state responsibilities for elderly persons.

Further reading

AHMAD, W. I. U. and ATKIN, K. (eds) (1996) *'Race' And Community Care*, Buckingham: Open University Press. Stimulating contributions on citizenship, family, disability, mental illness, social security and the voluntary sector.

MODOOD, T., BERTHOUD, R., LAKEY, J. *et al.* (eds) (1997) *Ethnic Minorities In Britain: Diversity and disadvantage*, London: Policy Studies Institute. Long awaited fourth national survey.

ALDERMAN, G. (1992) *Modern British Jewry*, Oxford: Clarendon Press. A highly readable, informative social analysis.

BOWES, A. and SIM, D. (eds) (1997) *Perspectives on Welfare: The experience of minority ethnic groups in Scotland*, Research in Ethnic Relations, Aldershot: Ashgate. Original research coverage of issues in Scottish housing, health and social care.

LAW, I. (1996) *Racism, Ethnicity and Social Policy*, Hemel Hempstead: Prentice Hall/Harvester Wheatsheaf. Explores policy and conceptual debates with the aid of primary research.

10
CITIZENSHIP, PARTICIPATION AND COMMUNITY CARE

Introduction

In Part II so far, we have examined issues relating to the users of community care. Given that the legislation's concern is to involve users, how does community care measure up to the underlying claims for enabling full citizenship? We have identified the key user groups as elderly persons, mentally distressed people, people with learning difficulties, and people with physical disabilities. This chapter will pose the question: To what extent have users benefited from the new emphasis upon citizenship and citizenship rights? It will be argued that full citizenship entails power, participation and involvement. Contemporary revival of interest in citizenship co-incided politically with attempts to redefine citizenship policy along the lines of market requirements. For users in community care, such a refocusing means legal advancements, new management strategies concerned with moving closer to user requirements, but little substantial progress in real citizenship rights or the recon-figuring of traditional power relationships. In advancing this argu-ment, the chapter will examine the developments in the concept of citizenship; the issue of rights; concepts of citizen as consumer and customer in the light of contemporary social and community policy; the incidence of participation, power and empowerment in community care, and the interrelationship between citizenship, participation and accountability; and finally, the relevance of com-munitarianism for the citizenship debate and community care.

Citizenship and social democracy

Citizenship as a concept has enjoyed a distinct revival over the past two decades. Some would argue that it has displaced social class by challenging the collective basis of traditional forms. For Barbalet (1988), citizenship 'defines those who are, and who are not, members of a common society' (ibid. p. 1). Clearly, it is a contested concept, which roughly divides between the liberal perspective and advocates of the communitarian position, since in the fullest sense of the word citizenship represents a complete attitude as well as a status (Oliver and Heater, 1994). While libertarian thought privileges the individual's citizenship rights, communitarian perspectives on active citizenship address duties owed to the individual. The issue of rights is at the heart of the current debate on the distribution of community care services, since the existence of rights elicits concomitant duties imposed upon the state to meet them. Alcock (1996) argues that the users of welfare services should be seen as citizens and not merely consumers. For example, as citizens they should have welfare rights, which in turn should be directly related to the need for empowerment and accountability in service delivery (Plant, 1988). Without the latter, user groups are too easily excluded from access to benefits (Alcock, 1996). As we have observed in preceding chapters, too often this has been the case with users of community care services.

Marshall's theory of rights

T. H. Marshall's *Citizenship and Social Class* (1950) set the parameters of the citizenship debate in this century. Modern citizen rights for Marshall have evolved in social democratic society, from civil (and legal) rights in contract theory in the later eighteenth and early nineteenth centuries, political rights in the nineteenth century (but only fully achieved in Britain in 1928), to the revival of social rights in the later nineteenth century but fully established in the British welfare state by the mid-twentieth century. For Marshall this was the lowest visible point of class distinction; relationships of contract were challenged by citizen status and the rule of market forces subordinated to social democracy's tenets of social justice.

But major contemporary critiques of Marshall suggest that his schema understates the continuing influences of private economic and corporate power in the twentieth-century welfare state, and evacuates social conflict and organised pressure from the smooth evolutionary unfolding of rights (Giddens, 1982; Taylor, D., 1989). Held (1984) advocates widening the debate to encompass questions raised by the new social movements' concerns with marginalisation from citizenship according to gender, 'race' and impairment. The crucial issues of economic power and social conflict are analysed below.

Community care, user involvement and citizenship

As a result of shifts in political power in Britain during the final decades of the twentieth century, rights and duties of citizens have been redefined in the areas of community care policies and legislation. What of user involvement and enhanced citizenship under such circumstances?

Community care legislation

As we saw in Chapter 4, the legislation came to encapsulate the reconstruction of welfare provision through expanded choice, rights and duties, empowerment, and greater responsiveness to 'customers' and the accountability of public services (Audit Commission, 1986; Department of Health, 1989). Section 46 of the NHS and Community Care Act 1990 outlines the role of the consultation of user groups in community care planning (Chapter 4). Subsequent policy guidance expected local authorities to consult voluntary organisations, housing agencies, health agencies, private agencies, carer groups and user groups. Nevertheless, the extent to which local authorities have integrated the involvement of user groups such as people with disabilities into the formulation of care plans is unclear.

Citizenship, duties and community care

Citizenship may also imply obligations as well as rights. But what of those in no position to meet 'obligations'? Many of the users and user groups within community care are unable to meet these, other than from the payments made by their family in the past. In areas such as long-term care for elderly people, payments spanning a lifetime are considered inadequate 'obligation' payment for the receipt of rights to care. This seems curious, given that a citizen's civil or political rights are conferred through one's citizen status without the associated duties or obligations (Plant, 1991). The social rights so confidently assumed by Marshall can no longer be taken for granted. The state's general duty appears to be one of providing in the collective sense, but not in the individual sense!

Notwithstanding the limits placed upon the state to meet its duties, caring in the community or by the community simply cannot rely upon the exercise of rights, but must incorporate a broader ethic of caring for and assisting others (Chapter 1). Citizenship needs to invoke a giving, and not only receiving, expressing an attitude and not just a status (Oliver and Heater, 1994) which entails action and involvement. This 'republican civic virtue' or communitarian perspective, is discussed later in greater detail. One of the problems we face, however, is that community care policies are implemented in the absence of recognising communitarian values. Our society denies full social citizenship in the case of people with disabilities for example. Far from expressing community, this becomes an exercise in communal exclusionism. Thus many people with disabilities have organised and actively seized their rights (see Chapter 6). Disability politics is indeed informed by the language of citizenship (Oliver, 1996; Lister, 1996; Barnes, 1997). But we may view the policy itself as ideological. Community care legislation outlines an important role for the voluntary sector and for active involvement of citizens; contracts in the voluntary sector act as a vehicle for stifling protest rather than supporting the seizure of citizen rights (Drake, 1996). It seems inconceivable too, for the state to adopt a non-interventionist stance on the attainment of citizen rights for user groups. Local government has a crucial role in providing resources, space and support for citizens: 'Where individuals are physically or mentally impaired, involvement must imply support and access' (Stewart, 1993, cited in Lister, 1996).

The citizen charter and consumerism

Much of the discourse on citizenship has been 'rewritten' by new right advocates of individual consumer rights. The Conservative

Government's Citizens' Charter in the early 1990s expressed the idea that individuals are consumers in possession of the power of choice, as in the market place. Accordingly, in the spirit of consumerism the Charter was closely allied to compulsory competitive tendering (CCT) in local government, based on the competitive contract system. Ideologically, the Charter's encouragement to act as individuals is tantamount to deterring collective political action. Although Oliver and Heater (1994) propose that such a Charter may add a dimension to the relations between citizen and state rather than subtract from citizenship, it appears that the equation of user groups in community care with consumers in the market renders this far from the case, for reasons articulated above.

Another cognate concept is that of citizen as 'customer', driven by the managerialist ideology underlying the structural shifts in health and social care services (Chapters 3 and 4). Managerialism has replaced the 'professional knowledge' model, with the aim of moving closer to the customer. Yet contrary to this individualised contractual relationship as a step along Marshall's evolutionary path of citizenship, we may well interpret it as a retreat to the seventeenth-century civil rights ideology of contract and individualism. Such ideology makes it all the more problematic in developing public support for a welfare state (Fraser and Gordon, 1994). The citizen as consumer and customer is defined in terms of personal responsibilities as consumer and customer as opposed to participant in collective action and involvement.

Finally, as we have discussed in Chapters 3 and 4, purchasers and providers in health and social care must operate within the framework of a mixed economy and quasi-markets intended to express individual requirements, an environment which reinforces market individualism, the polarity of communitarianism or civic republicanism. The implicit requirement of socially vulnerable user groups to meet obligations and the absence of any state duty to provide for individuals raise ethical questions. By the same token, the state's concentration on rights denies the communitarian impulse to intervene and provide for active citizenship and involvement. Contemporary policy interpretations of citizenship would seem more engaged with consumer and customer rights for services purchased in the quasi-markets, which leads us to consider the relationships between participation and power.

Participation, power and empowerment in community care

Not only does the legislation and guidance imply a form of citizenship; it also indicates a reordering of power relationships by the 'empowerment' of users. But are power relationships being transformed to the advantage of the user groups? Citizenship may bring more participation, but does not necessarily enhance power enjoyed by these groups. On the contrary, it will be argued that participation in community and community care decisions is harder to achieve for those groups technically 'dependent' on the policies. If anything, the protest movements referred to earlier have effected greater shifts in power relationships than have any formal consultation procedures.

Power and empowerment

What is empowerment? It is a term in the 'community care' discourse which, like 'community', is clothed in an ambiguity of meaning and can involve the empowering of others while not giving up one's own power (Gomm, 1993). Strictly speaking, one needs to talk in terms of the degree of empowerment achieved by user groups. Three major approaches to attaining empowerment have been delineated: empowerment through 'exit'; empowerment through 'voice'; and empowerment through 'rights' (Taylor *et al.*, 1995).

The 'exit' model assumes that with the development of welfare mix and the 'marketisation' of health and social care services, users may 'shop around' in planning for their future needs, and thus boast the power to withdraw from purchasing a service. But how many users are in a position of such 'consumer sovereignty' among disabled or elderly users of services, given the low average income levels? Empowerment by 'voice' refers to the opportunities for placing pressures on the providers through user committees or similar forums, or influencing care managers in the formation of care 'packages' and type of delivery. Yet in such a process much depends upon the degree to which purchasers, providers and care managers are prepared to share power with users.

How much power can user groups exert by being consulted? Research has shown that although more consultation materialised in the 1990s than in the previous decade, user involvement was not central in decision making: '[Power] was still effectively located within large-scale welfare bureaucracies.' By the middle of the 1990s, 'the size of the task implied by developing community care as an empowering service option was perhaps more evident than it had been when the architects of the 1990 Act were doing their work' (Barnes, 1997, p. 99).

Empowerment through 'rights' is the third key mode of empowerment, and, as we have noted earlier, it is a position accepted by the disability movement for obtaining recognition of full citizenship for disabled people. We have also seen (Chapter 6) how concerted pressure from the disability movement through the courts initially won the legal right for assessed needs to be met by the providing authority, regardless of resources (although the verdict was subsequently overturned). While 'empowerment' *per se* should not be dismissed, since it does offer all kinds of potential, it is frequently utilised as justification and legitimation for continued professional power and control, more of a 'regulatory' empowerment (Fawcett and Featherstone, 1996, p. 54). It is empowerment as containment, collusion, and a depoliticising of action (Humphreys, 1996). Again, this brings into question whether participation means power. Participation as a valid exercise is marginalised, along with the effectiveness of user groups without wider accompanying socio-economic structural changes (Croft and Beresford, 1992).

And what of accountability? If service users have a right of 'voice' over services in general, then they ought to receive information on their availability and their performance; the services should, in other words, be accountable to the users. The more that restructured services become local, and tender choice (as in the health service), then the more such accountability should be operating at the local level. Accountability ought no longer to be seen as purely applicable to the national level. Current democratic accountability has to be public and local (Daly, 1996). And accountability demands dialogue between purchasers, providers and user groups. Such a concept threatens the power of professionals, and may cause discomfort to the latter. User groups have detected a shift in power and opportunities in planning forums to make public services accountable through more frequent contact and dialogue with purchasers and providers (Barnes, 1997). Although the Department of

Health has issued guidance (e.g. 'Local Voices') and directives for greater openness on the part of health trusts, health authorities and GP family health authorities (now amalgamated with health authorities), a local democratic deficit results due to the proliferation of non-elected bodies (quangos) (Daly, 1996). Local citizens have been distanced and their local councillors have less chance to intervene, given the new 'enabling' role of local authorities, and the introduction of CCT and contract culture (Hill, 1994). To cite the Commission on Social Justice: 'Only if accountability can be strengthened will people gain rights, not merely as customers but as citizens' (Borrie, 1994, p. 352).

Summarising the relationship between participation, empowerment and power, the widely invoked term empowerment remains ambiguous. Exit by 'voice' is subject to professional managers' agreement, consultation which is improving but not fully involving, and 'rights' which are legalised and individualised. Participation does not necessarily serve to empower. Decentralisation of services may suggest a more direct and accessible accountability to user groups, yet the rise of quangos and the redefinition of local authority functions has left a local gap in accountability. The next section considers the growing contribution of communitarianism to the citizenship and participation debate.

Citizenship, community and communitarianism

It ought to be apparent by now that the relationships between community and the market-driven definitions of citizenship are rather strained. Communitarian philosophy proposes that the conflict is irresolvable unless one refutes the notion of individuals exercising rights or responsibilities divorced from collective common purpose. An increased receptivity to communitarian ideas has surfaced with the related anxieties over the consequences of individualistic behaviour.

The philosophical communitarians

A small group of North American academic philosophers is instrumental in renewing public interest in communitarian philosophies which stand in the classical Judaeo-Christian, Greek and Roman and Marxist traditions. In a climate of market-orientated social policy making, and through their pointed debates with liberal philosopher John Rawls (1974) and the more right-wing Robert Nozick (1974), they have vociforously countered the contemporary passion for individual citizenship rights in the United States, re-asserting human beings' essential communal nature and the inviol-ability of social duties and responsibilities. Alasdair MacIntyre (1985) deems that the community should serve a moral purpose in laying out agreed guidelines and virtues for human action, such as the importance of friendship for the communal form of life. Charles Taylor (1989) promotes the significance of community and commitment within a social framework. If we accept this position, we may understand that a contract culture posited on the negotia-tion of individual advantage is antithetical to such commitment.

Michael Sandel (1982, 1992) points to the centrality of parti-cipation in refining one's sense of identity and belonging as citizens to a particular community or republic. The relevance of this perspective to users of community care is evident. People with disabilities, for instance, unable to participate fully in many activities of communities which deny them proper access, have formed new communities of identity. Michael Walzer (1983) argues that community and social meaning has to be prioritised above the individual in deciding on how goods and services are to be allocated. Various goods and services such as health and social care must not be classified as subject to the 'ability to pay' criterion even in the context of capitalist markets. One might add that quasi-markets and competitive values provide the framework for citizens' entitlements under community care in Britain; the 'community' in this case is not automatically fettered to caring but is paired with concepts of devolved power and enhanced service delivery (Peters and Marshall, 1996).

Etzioni's new communitarianism

Amatai Etzioni's new communitarianism stems from a similar disquiet with the failure of community, but is more grounded in organised community 'projects'. His *Spirit of Community* (Etzioni, 1993) rejects the narrow preoccupation with rights and calls for a broader concern with obligations. New communitarianism advo-cates more of balance between the assertion of a public interest (as distinct from political sectional interests) and individual concerns and rights, urging the recognition of the citizen's prime duties to the community. More specifically, Etzioni's programme for the 'remoralisation of society' concentrates on the areas of education, family and parenting, law and order, and neighbourhood, holding the voluntary sector as playing a leading role in forging the viable community. Etzioni portrays each of these areas of social life as in a state of crisis – new moral attitudes must be the order of the day, faced with the breakdown of family and communal values, ideas of a 'moral code' and a fragmenting of the traditional left–right political persuasion appeal to large sections of both New Right and Democrat Americans. Indeed, the relevance of the ideas to local community and direct accountability has also attracted British political activists and 'New Labour', navigating a route between collectivism and individualism (Mulgan, 1997). For example, in the Birmingham inner-city Balsall Heath area, community activist Dick Atkinson (1994) promotes the development of rank-and-file projects which build community from the bottom upwards, based upon the strengthening of family, schooling and work.

Critiques of communitarianism

Communitarianism in itself, however, is open to criticism. Opposition to philosophical communitarianism points to the romanticising of past communities; a substantial gap exists between the prescriptions for the good society and the actual environment of the model communitarian societies. Furthermore, the assumptions made of such idealised communities, for example the participative Greek democracy, evade the oppressive aspects of their economic and social structures for women. In the case of the allegedly more practical new communitarianism, much of its force stems from the moral statements for changing community, with no real attempt to connect with the realities of unequal power relationships and the prerequisites for changing these structures. As with the 'silence' from the philosophical school, new communitarianism's restatement of traditional family structures and values is in danger of reinforcing the oppression of women in the community (Chapter 8). It pays no attention to the community of identity born out of a sense of common oppression (Friedman, 1992), as with, for instance, the Disability Movement. New communitarianism's foundational assumptions and prescriptions for returning to the traditional family, while serving to justify community care policy, implicitly exclude women from participation in the citizen body because of their caring capacities (Kingdom, 1996).

Communitarianism and community care

For both constituents of the term to be meaningful, community care must be founded on communitarian values that privilege caring and confine the criterion of 'ability to pay' to appropriate commodities. Communitarianism as a philosophy supplies the rationale for all to participate as citizens in decisions for allocating goods and services. But parity in participation and outcomes requires parity in power relationships and access to material resources. Such egalitarianism and the relegation of 'ability to pay' demands the supportive role of the state rather than the unequalising forces of the market place.

New communitarianism strongly advocates the voluntary sector as the most likely arena in which citizen participation may flourish. Hirst's 'associationism' (1994) supports the idea of voluntary organisations' greater responsiveness compared with bureaucratic behaviour, and their superior effectiveness in engaging citizens and users. However, as we have noted, the operation of the quasi-markets, by steering voluntary organisations into 'contract' culture, threatens the continuation of voluntary organisations, and in so doing, marginalises user groups such as those in mental health or the African-Caribbean organisations whose participation is expressed most readily within the voluntary sector. If community care, then, is to fully reflect communitarian values, further radical changes in power and access to resources are necessary, in that market procedures have effectively distanced user groups from the 'constituent' communities.

Conclusion

This chapter has assessed the extent of user involvement and empowerment resulting from community care policies. It has also examined how communitarianism potentially posed an ideological alternative to consumerism. Citizenship may have returned to the political agenda with the emphasis on rights and the ostensible devaluation of social-class affiliations, but in the light of the overall marginalising effects of quasi-markets evidence is lacking to show that the new consumerist citizenship actually empowers community care user groups. While various modes of empowerment are available for user groups, the practical outcomes are less than satisfactory, given the maintenance of control by managers and the distorting impacts of market relationships which atomise individuals. Decentralisation may well hint at an increased potential for direct accountability to users at the local level, yet up to now this has been deflected by the institution of non-elected bodies which manage to bypass social democratic processes. Direct accountability is also displaced by purchaser:provider procedures which result in the user becoming a third party onlooker. The brand of 'citizenship' offered by community care coexists uneasily with the communitarian scenario of citizens deeply involved in the community's decision-making framework and power structures. 'Community' in the latter sense seems at odds with consumerist citizenship. Certainly, new communitarianism's advocacy of the traditional family structure and its implied minimal state support for female carers is a serious flaw in this modern critique of community policies. Yet without the recognition of some form of communitiarian values, community care stands as a contradiction in terms.

Further reading

BARNES, M. (1997) *Care, Communities and Citizens*, London: Longman. A review of research and debates on local citizenship.

HUMPHREYS, B. (ed.) (1996) *Critical Perspectives On Empowerment*, Birmingham: Venture Press. A succinct exploration of the concept as applied to caring, disability, sexuality, poverty and social work.

RAMCHARAN, P., ROBERTS, G., GRANT, G. and BORLAND, J. (eds) (1997) *Empowerment in Everyday Life: Learning disability*, London: Jessica Kingsley. A collection focusing on the exclusion from social and political participation of people with learning difficulties.

ETZIONI, A. (ed.) (1995) *New Communitarian Thinking: Persons, virtues, institutions, and communities*, Charlottesville, Va.: University of Virginia Press. Essays on community, democracy and citizenship.

11
SUMMARY AND CONCLUSIONS

This book has aimed to convey the complexities of community care policy by analysing the diverse elements of community care. It set out to chart the broad changes in community in modern Britain, and situate them in the context of social policy and the overarching ideological environment. This was in order to accurately locate the crucial interrelationships between community care, ideology and social policy, and to identify key processes and legislation transforming decision-making structures in community care. Finally, it has sought to identify and assess major issues of policy and institutional changes, and their respective impacts upon community care user groups.

Contemporary community care issues echo earlier institutional responses to nineteenth-century population growth and the escalating needs of user groups who rarely encountered humane treatment. Clearly, the voluntary sector has become a permanent feature since the previous century; the state's own role has fluctuated to some extent with the political perspectives of the ruling government but more so with the ruling paradigm of an epoch, irrespective of political party affiliation. One might conjecture that Britain's social policy underwent its first *real* paradigm shift at the mid-point of the present century with the implementation of the welfare state, and its second with the ascendancy of New Right Thatcherite thinking, now likely to endure into the next century.

The NHS and Community Care Act 1990 and related government directives leave little doubt as to the integral connection of health policy with community care. Policy changes in the health and social services are now driven in this sense by the same motor. Health care reforms are of course ideological and mirror the principal transitions in the social services – the initiation of a purchaser:provider split, the focus on primary care and the promotion of GP fund-holding practices, and the inculcation of overt competitive behaviour between health trusts. Changes are now pending in the health service with respect to the removal of GP fund-holding, but with similar alternatives, while the new Labour Government White Paper proposals emerging at the end of 1997 for the removal of internal markets will not take effect until the latter part of the next decade. The contemporary NHS blueprint was informed by an ideology of managerialism and constituent efficiency criteria prioritising cost minimisation. A preoccupation with costs and responsibility for long-term health care for an expanding elderly population will bind health care to community care for many years ahead. But no solution is viable without resources and without durable mechanisms for collaboration with social care agencies; this evidently persists as a key problem that authorities will need to rectify over the coming period. Mental health services decentralisation, coupled with poor institutional coordination, poses a particularly serious policy hiatus. The Conservative Government's failure to deal with this crucial area of community care has left a thorny legacy for the new Labour Government to grasp.

Major restructuring of social services is rationalised by a managerialist philosophy which prioritises organisational goals. Moreover, the new contract culture not only reformulates the *raison d'être* of social services, but has transposed inherently 'not for profit' voluntary bodies into precariously supported state businesses. Care becomes management, with local authorities now managing the activities of contractors and mediating with clients as consumers. Consequently, the duties of the social worker are now redefined, suggesting serious deskilling and a worsening of already stressful working conditions because of rapidly diminishing resources.

Social policy processes, as with economic restructuring, have become increasingly globalised. The new paradigm and the subsequent reforms in community care are manifestly not unique to Britain, with comparable economies undergoing their own sets of health reforms which embody managerialism, quality and efficiency criteria, decentralised structures and quasi-market competition. This implies that any analysis of British social policy and community care strategies must integrate such globalising tendencies as post-Fordism, as well as more localised political forces.

Recipients of care services have been generally neglected by a community care literature more intent on addressing the technical administrative imperatives that arise out of formal legislation. Yet user groups in community care are more subject to social exclusion than the population at large, the full explanation of which entails understanding the impacts of social class, gender and ethnicity in tandem with the ideological underpinnings of social policy. It is important to note, however, that while the marginalisation of such social groups may well cut across social class in certain circumstances – for example, people with learning disabilities – the effects of social class are overarching, compounding difficulties experienced by certain groups in need of community care. This may appear self-evident in the light of the analysis throughout the book, but so much sociological policy and cultural commentary on contemporary western society has wrongly assumed that class divisions are no longer significant. ('We're all consumers now' might be an apt post-modernist sound bite representing this position.) The users of community care largely comprise those who have been economically and socially excluded. These include people with mental health difficulties rendered homeless, people with disabilities and elderly people.

Elderly people are high on the community care policy agenda, given their rising numbers, although it is certainly the case that many old people never require care. Old people bear the brunt of the organisational health:social care divide, because of the cost implications of long-term care. Often they suffer inappropriate care, victims of a historical social and institutional ageism exacerbated by financial hardship for those who must depend on a basic pension. The close relationship between poverty and old age, especially for economically marginalised women, is a serious cause for concern. Here, at least, the schism of economic and social policy is a nonsense.

We may ascribe the sharpened profile of disabled people in community care much more to organisational power and collective strength than to official bureaucratic directives. Disability groups' raised consciousness has steered this new movement, increasingly influential in invoking civil rights and citizenship, beyond the strict parameters of formal participation in community care forums. The poor synchronisation between housing and community care policies simultaneous with the growth of homelessness among mentally disturbed people underscores the essential nature of a housing policy inexplicably disregarded during the initial period of the contemporary community care reforms. A wholesale reduction in the social housing stock is now a major hindrance to successful local institutional support for users living in the community. While the supply of social housing is now in the hands of housing associations, their capacity to build remains highly dependent on state (Housing Corporation) funding.

But policy must also tackle the issue of how to balance the claims to citizenship rights of mentally ill homeless persons against the public's need for physical safety and state protection. Both homelessness and violence embody a legacy of treating deinstitutionalisation as panacea for consistent mental health care, in the absence of adequate staffing and resourcing.

Women are still the foundation of informal care, an army of unpaid labour whose position is assiduously justifed by the discourse of familialism. Having said this, it is clear that women are not simply bludgeoned into informal family caring; the motives are complex and many women care voluntarily. Yet women caring in the community are hampered by inhospitable community environments, plus their own poverty and poor health which may arise from years of intensive caring. Women are not only carers, however. The belief that this is their only role subjugates the need for autonomy among those women who are being cared for.

Minority ethnic groups, including African-Caribbeans and Asians, accustomed sufferers of racism in one form or another, experience discriminatory practice in community care through their exposure to the insensitivities of institutional services. 'White' institutions adopt familiar assumptions that minority group elders are either returning to their original homeland or that their 'own' communities or families will look after them. Yet, in effect, a multiplicity of practices and tendencies operates in, for example, the Chinese, African-Caribbean and Jewish communities.

Contemporary community care legislation pays considerable attention to 'empowerment' and the availability of wider choices on the 'consumerist' model of policy making. But in terms of outcome, the formal mechanisms for participation do not necessarily empower. New 'citizenship', by dint of its commercial context, supplants political citizenship with consumerist 'choice', which simultaneously acts as a flexible instrument of control for new public sector management. We may well perceive communitarian-ism as an antidote to market and managerialist ideology: an expression of public unease at an ostensible crumbling of the 'social cement'. Caring *by* the community, on the other hand, implies a tangible community, which consumerist individualism has seriously damaged. In this respect, the adoption of the quasi-market is antithetical to a communally based culture. It is also hard to see how friendship and neighbourhood networks are prepared or competent for providing regular caring. In the last analysis, women (and a few men) in the household *are* the community, frequently caring with minimal support.

Community care policy has to be evaluated and understood in relation to ideological and social policy imperatives in historical context. For example, the period of the classic welfare state and collectivist state provision, where strong comprehensive institutions were charged with meeting a host of universal demands, meant community care *in* the community as opposed to care *by* the com-munity, yet the family care (basically carried out by women) was on a large scale and officially justified through the Beveridge philo-sophy. In this latter respect, it is hard to detect a fundamental change in government philosophy or policy. Community care policy has been critical in relocating social policy's centre of gravity from the public to the private sphere. The eighteen years of Thatcherite policies evinced a social paradigmatic shift. One might venture that, given global post-modernist tendencies towards the political centre, it is expected to survive through the early years of the twenty-first century. Managerialism is an essential ideological component of the ruling paradigm which today not only dominates the running of social and health services, but also the new public sector as a whole, from education through to housing and other arms of local government, a 'managerialist state' which strives to curb traditional professional power. As the book has attempted to show, managerialism's discourse of values may yield certain cor-porate advantages within particular circumstances, but we have to question whether they are realisable or even desirable in the care domain, or indeed wherever social relations as distinct from material transactions are paramount.

Practical policy issues and strategic level considerations, which reflect the ideological reorientations in social policy, then face community care policy makers. Community care policy must deliver quality accommodation for mentally distressed people who are bewildered by closure of the large hospitals. The purchaser:provider split would seem better suited for improving service efficiency in the context of quasi-markets, but where do these fit with the aims of community care legislation to empower users of services? Again, with the increase in contracting, welfare pluralism accords an elevated position to voluntary bodies in the independent sector, but it is arguable whether state support adequately equips them to professionalise their operations.

Ineffective collaboration is a recurrent problem. Following the 'faulty start' at the beginning of the 1990s, local authorities may claim improvements in collaborative arrangements. Yet elderly people seem caught in a financial pincer movement between health and social care services. The plight of mental health sufferers too has deteriorated because of inadequate arrangements between community care bodies and housing authorities. At the time of writing, no genuine alternative had been offered by the new government, although it had flagged up a reversal of policy for hospitalised mentally ill patients.

One returns full circle to the 'community' component of community care. Care policies are locally focused, but the user groups are ostensibly trapped in a vacuum of the localised community. In the non-spatial, relational sense however, community may have been preserved among self-organised user groups. But with the change of government, what is the status of the market/managerialist paradigm at the late twentieth century as it relates to community care? Given the centre-right political position of New Labour, the new government is engaged in a refashioning of the Thatcherite paradigm as opposed to its overthrow; welfare mix serves as the basis of health and social policies. There is already a declared intention to relegate the significance of competition in the public sector with, for example, an early questioning of compulsory competitive tendering for local government servicing. New Labour's health service strategy over the next few years is to flatten public expenditure, but it is also prepared to eventually remove the GP fund-holding system, according to the 1997 comprehensive review and White Paper on the NHS. Yet in spite of Labour's move to replace the 1990s model of the GP fund-holding practice, it holds on to the principle of the purchaser:provider distinction. Substantial problems will still be encountered in creating a viable financial programme for long-term care that takes into account the economic position of millions of elderly people, yet the new government has displayed few signs of progress in tackling the issue. Whereas Labour has seemingly rejected the option of private insurance, it is slow to act. Age Concern estimated in1997 that positive decisions were unlikely for at least another five years. In the meantime, Labour announced a long-term care charter and Royal Commission for the future. Local panels were instituted for overseeing local health authority–social services agreements. It is striking that the private insurance companies themselves have shown reluctance to enter the long-term care insurance market, cognisant that only one in six of the population can afford the average £50,000 cost of care. Long-term care for elderly people stands as a further great challenge for New Labour.

New Labour communicates a plausible concern for the revitalisation of downtrodden communities, not least by way of its job creation programmes. In many respects, Tony Blair's Christian socialism resembles Etzioni's new communitarianism, a replacement of neo-liberal individualism as the basis for future community care policy. Yet the uncritical championing of familialism normalises the acceptability of large-scale unpaid informal caring by women. New communitarianism construes 'community' as complementary to the market instead of replacing it. Labour's preparedness to intervene in social issues through the state mechanisms is unmistakably greater than that of the last Conservative government, but it is proving an equivocal intervention. Reliance upon charitable sources for funding community care is as marked as ever. One may speculate whether the employment-focused urban regeneration strategy, coupled with a communitarian philosophy, will ensure that more government attention is paid to communities *per se*. Certainly, the new devolution of government is an encouragement for dovetailing health, social care and housing plans at a more local level. Unfortunately, the government's decisions to cut social security benefits for lone parents and disability benefits signifies a triumph of the market paradigm. They reflect New Labour's tentativeness in challenging big business pressures for reduced social expenditure. In the meantime, inadequate community care for millions will prove Britain's most obstinate social policy predicament unless the causes of social marginalisation are rigorously confronted.

BIBLIOGRAPHY

ABBERLEY, P. (1993) 'Disabled people and "normality"', in J. Swain, V. Finklestein, S. French and M. Oliver (eds), *Disabling Barriers – Enabling Environments*, London: Sage

ABERCROMBIE, N., WARDE, A., SOOTHILL, K., URRY, J. and WALBY, S. (eds) (1994) *Contemporary British Society*, 2nd edn, Cambridge: Polity

AHMAD, W. I. (ed.) (1993) *'Race' And Health In Contemporary Britain*, Buckingham: Open University Press

AHMAD, W. I. (1996) 'Family obligations and social change among Asian communities', in W. I. Ahmad and K. Atkin (eds) (1996), *'Race' and Community Care*, Buckingham: Open University Press

AHMAD, W. I. and ATKIN, K. (eds) (1996), *'Race' and Community Care*, Buckingham: Open University Press

ALASZEWSKI, A. and WUN, W. L. (1994) 'Residential services', in N. Malin (ed.) *Implementing Community Care*, Buckingham: Open University Press

ALBER, J. (1992) *Older People in Europe: Social and economic policies: National Report Germany*, Konstanz: University of Konstanz

ALBER, J. (1993) 'Health and social services', in A. Walker, J. Alber and A-M. Guillemard (eds), *Older People in Europe: Social and economic policies*, Brussels: Commission of the European Communities

ALBER, J. (1995) 'A framework for the comparative study of social services', *Journal of European Social Policy*, **5** (2), 113–49

ALCOCK, P. (1996) *Social Policy In Britain: Themes and issues*, London: Macmillan

ALDERMAN, G. (1992) *Modern British Jewry*, Oxford: Clarendon Press

ALDRIDGE, J. and BECKER, S. (1996) 'Disability rights and the denial of young carers: the dangers of zero-sum arguments', *Critical Social Policy*, **48**, 55–76

ALLEN, D. (1996) 'Women on the edge', *Community Care*, 5–11 December

ALLEN, I., HOGG, O. and PEACE, S. (1992) *Elderly People: Choice, participation and satisfaction*, London: Policy Studies Institute

211

ALLSOP, J. (1994) *Health Policy and the NHS Towards 2000*, London: Longman

ANDERSON, B. (1991) *Imagined Communities*, London: Verso

ANTTONEN, A. and SIPILA, J. (1996) 'European social care services: is it possible to identify models?', *Journal of European Social Policy*, **6** (2), 87–100

ARBER, S., GILBERT, G. N. and EVANDROU, M. (1988) 'Gender, household composition and receipt of domiciliary services by elderly disabled people', *Journal of Social Policy*, **17**, 153–75

ARBER, S. and GINN, J. (1989) 'Men: the forgotten carers', *Sociology*, **23** (1), 111–18

ARBER, S. and GINN, J. (1991) *Gender and Later Life*, London: Sage

ARBER, S. and GINN, J. (eds) (1995) *Connecting Gender and Ageing: A sociological approach*, Buckingham: Open University Press

ASHTON, T. (1995) 'From evolution to revolution: restructuring the New Zealand health system', in D. Seedhouse (ed.), *Reforming Health Care: The philosophy and practice of international health reform*, Chichester: Wiley

ATKIN, K. (1996) 'An opportunity for change: voluntary sector provision in a mixed economy of care', in W. I. Ahmad and K. Atkin (eds), *'Race' and Community Care*, Buckingham: Open University Press

ATKIN, K. and ROLLINGS, J. (1996) 'Looking after their own? Family care-giving among Asian and Afro-Caribbean communities', in W. I. Ahmad and K. Atkin (eds), *'Race' And Community Care*, Buckingham: Open University Press

ATKINSON, D. (1994) *The Common Sense of Identity*, London: Demos

AUDIT COMMISSION (1986) *Making a Reality of Community Care*, London: HMSO

AUDIT COMMISSION (1996) *What the Doctor Ordered: A study of GP fundholders in England and Wales*, London: HMSO

AUSTIN, R. (1996) 'Tangled web', *Community Care*, 7–13 March

BAGGULEY, P. (1994) 'Prisoners of the Beveridge dream? The political mobilisation of the poor against contemporary welfare regimes', in R. Burrows and B. Loader (eds), *Towards A Post-Fordist Welfare State?*, London: Routledge

BALDOCK, J. and UNGERSON, C. (1991) ' "What d'ya want if you don' want money?" – a feminist critique of "paid volunteering" ', in M. Maclean and D. Groves (eds), *Women's Issues In Social Policy*, London: Routledge

BALDWIN, S. (1994) 'The need for care in later life: social protection for older people and family care givers', in S. Baldwin and J. Falkingham (eds), *Social Security and Social Change: New challenges to the Beveridge model*, Hemel Hempstead: Harvester Wheatsheaf

BALDWIN, S. and LUNT, N. (1996a) *Charging Ahead: Local authority charging policies for community care*, York: Joseph Rowntree Foundation/Policy Press

BALDWIN, S. and LUNT, N. (1996b) 'Hard charging', *Community Care*, 13–19 June, 28–9

BALDWIN, S. and TWIGG, J. (1991) 'Women and community care: reflections on a debate', in M. Maclean and D. Groves (eds), *Women's Issues In Social Policy*, London: Routledge

BANNERMAN, L. and ROBERTSON, B. (1996) 'Care management: a manager's perspective', in C. Clark and I. Lapsley (eds), *Planning and Costing Community Care*, Research Highlights in Social Work no. 27, London: Jessica Kingsley

BARBALET, J. (1988) *Citizenship*, Buckingham: Open University Press

BARHAM, P. (1992) *Closing The Asylum: The mental patient in modern society*, Harmondsworth: Penguin

BARKER, R. (1997) *Political Ideas In Modern Britain: In and after the 20th century*, 2nd edn, London: Routledge

BARNES, C. (1992) 'Institutional discrimination against disabled people and the campaign for anti-discrimination legislation', *Critical Social Policy*, **34**, 5–22

BARNES, C. (1994) *Disabled People in Britain and Discrimination*, 2nd rev. repr., London: Hurst

BARNES, M. (1997) *Care, Communities and Citizens*, London: Longman

BARTON, L. (1993) 'The struggle for citizenship: the case of disabled people', *Disability, Handicap and Society*, **8** (3), 235–48

BEAN, P. and MOUNSER, P. (1993) *Discharged From Mental Hospitals*, London: Macmillan

BEAUCHAMP, D. E. and AMBROSE, P. M. (1994) 'Managing the contradictions in the Clinton health plan', in P. Vaillancourt Rosenau (ed.), *Health Care Reform In The Nineties*, London: Sage

BEAZLEY, M. (1994) 'Measuring service quality', in N. Malin (ed.), *Implementing Community Care*, Buckingham: Open University Press

BEGUM, N. (1992) 'Doubly disabled', *Community Care*, September

BEGUM, N. (1994) 'Optimism, pessimism and care management: the impact of community care policies', in N. Begum, M. Hill and A. Stevens (eds), *Reflections: Views of black disabled people on their lives and community care*, London: CCETSW

BEGUM, N. (1995) 'Care management from an anti-racist perspective', *Social Care Research Findings*, **65**, York: Joseph Rowntree Foundation

BEGUM, W. (1990) *Burden of Gratitude: Women with disabilities receiving personal care*, Coventry: University of Warwick

BELL, C. and NEWBY, H. (1971) *Community Studies: An introduction to the sociology of the local community*, London: Allen & Unwin

BELLAMY, R. (1993) 'Liberalism', in R. Eatwell and A. Wright (eds), *Contemporary Political Ideologies*, London: Pinter

BENNET, G. and KINGSTON, P. (1993) *Elder Abuse: Concepts, theories and interventions*, London: Chapman & Hall

BENZEVAL, M. (1997) 'Health', in A. Walker and C. Walker (eds), *Britain Divided: The growth of social exclusion in the 1980s and 1990s*, London: CPAG

BERMAN, M. (1983) *All That Is Solid Melts Into Air: The experience of modernity*, London: Verso

BEURET, K. (1991) 'Women and transport', in M. Maclean and D. Groves (eds), *Women's Issues In Social Policy*, London: Routledge

BEWLEY, C. and GLENDENNING, C. (1994) 'Representing the views of disabled people in community care planning', *Disability and Society*, **9** (3), 301–14

BIGGS, S. (1993) *Understanding Ageing: Images, attitudes and professional practice*, Buckingham: Open University Press

BLAKEMORE, K. and BONEHAM, M. (1994) *Age, Race and Ethnicity: A comparative approach*, Buckingham: Open University Press

BLAKEMORE, K. and DRAKE, R. (1996) *Understanding Equal Opportunity Policies*, Hemel Hempstead: Prentice Hall/Harvester Wheatsheaf

BLAND, R. (1994a) 'EPIC – A Scottish Case Management Experiment', in M. Titterton (ed.), *Caring for People in the Community*, London: Jessica Kingsley

BLAND, R. (1994b) 'The interdisciplinary assessment of need in community care', in R. Davidson and S. Hunter (eds), *Community Care In Practice*, London: Batsford

BOND, J., COLEMAN, P. and PEACE, S. (eds) (1993) *Ageing and Society*, London: Sage

BORNAT, J. (1993) 'Representations of community', in J. Bornat, C. Pereira, D. Pilgrim and F. Williams (eds), *Community Care: A Reader*, London: Macmillan

BORNAT, J., PEREIRA, C., PILGRIM, D., and WILLIAMS, F. (eds) (1993) *Community Care: A reader*, London: Macmillan

BORNAT, J., PHILLIPSON, C. and WARD, S. (1985) *A Manifesto For Old Age*, London: Pluto

BORRIE, G./Commission on Social Justice (1994) *Social Justice: Strategies for national renewal*, London: Vintage

BRADLEY, J. and SUTHERLAND, V. (1995) 'Occupational stress in social services: a comparison of social workers and home help staff', *British Journal of Social Work*, **25** (3), 313–32

BRADSHAW, J. (1977) 'The concept of social need', in M. Fitzgerald, P. Halmos, J. Muncie and D. Zeldin (eds), *Welfare in Action*, London: RKP

BRANDON, D. (1995) 'Peer support and advocacy: international comparisons and developments', in R. Jack (ed.), *Empowerment in Community Care*, London: Chapman & Hall

BRAYBON, J. (1996) 'Fear of the fall-out factor', *Guardian*, 27 November, 'Society' supplement

BRENTON, M. (1985) *The Voluntary Sector in British Social Services*, London: Longman

BRINDLE, D. (1996a) 'Shaky step forward', *Guardian*, 27 November, 'Society' supplement

BRINDLE, D. (1996b) 'Lack of GPs shows North–South divide', *Guardian*, 4 May

BROOKS, E. R., ZUNIGA, M. and PENN, N. E. (1995) 'The decline of public mental health in the United States', in C. V. Willie, P. Perri-Rieker, B. M. Kramer and B. S. Brown (eds), *Mental Health, Racism and Sexism*, London: Taylor & Francis

BROWN, G. W. and HARRIS, T. (1978) *Social Origins of Depression: A study of psychiatric disorder in women*, London: Tavistock

BROWN, J. (1994) 'The caring professions', in N. Malin (ed.), *Implementing Community Care*, Buckingham: Open University Press

BROWN, M. and PAYNE, S. (1994) *Introduction to Social Administration in Britain*, 7th edn, London: Unwin Hyman

BRYAN, B., DALZIE, S. and SCAFE, S. (1985) *The Heat of the Race: Black women's lives in Britain*, London: Virago

BRYSON, L. (1992) *Welfare and the State*, London: Macmillan

BULMER, M. (1987) *The Social Bases of Community Care*, London: Allen & Unwin

BULMER, M., LEWIS, J. and PICHAUD, D. (eds) (1989) *The Goals of Social Policy*, London: Unwin Hyman

BUTCHER, H., GLEN, A., HENDERSON, P. and SMITH, J. (1993) *Community And Public Policy*, London: Pluto

BUTLER, N., (1987) 'Ageism', in G. L. Maddox (ed.), *Encyclopaedia of Aging*, New York: Springer

BUTT, J. and MIRZA, K. (1996) *Social Care and Black Communities: A review of recent research studies*, London: HMSO

BYTHEWAY, W. and JOHNSON, J. (1990) 'On defining ageism', *Critical Social Policy*, **29**, 27–39

CAHILL, M. (1994) *New Social Policy*, Oxford: Blackwell

CAIN, H. and YUVAL-DAVIS, N. (1990) 'The "equal opportunities community" and the anti-racist struggle', *Critical Social Policy*, **29**, 5–26

CAMPBELL, D. (1996) 'The price of terror', *Guardian*, 10 December

CARLISLE, D. (1996) 'Friends in need', *Community Care*, 20–26 June, 29

CARPENTER, M. (1994) *Normality is Hard Work: Trade unions and the politics of community care*, London: Lawrence & Wishart

CARTER, T. and NASH, C. (1995) 'Pensioners' forums: a voice for older people', in R. Jack (ed.), *Empowerment in Community Care*, London: Chapman & Hall

CASHMORE, E. (1996) *Dictionary of Race and Ethnic Relations*, 4th edn, London: Routledge

CASSAM, E. and GUPTA, H. (1992) *Quality Assurance for Social Care Agencies*, London: Longman

CAUGHEY, J. (1996) 'Psychological distress in staff of a social services district office: a pilot study', *British Journal of Social Work*, June, **26** (3), 389–98

CCETSW (1995) *Assuring Quality in the Diploma in Social Work-1: Rules and requirements for the DipSW*, rev. edn, London: CCETSW

CERVI, B. (1996) 'Cut to fit', *Community Care*, 18–24 April, 18–19

CHADDA, D. (1996) 'Potential difference', *Health Service Journal*, 30 May, 7

CHADWICK, A. (1996) 'Knowledge, power and the Disability Discrimination Bill', *Disability and Society*, **11** (1), 25–40

CHALLIS, D. (1994a) 'Case management: a review of UK developments and issues', in M. Titterton (ed.), *Caring for People in the Community*, London: Jessica Kingsley

CHALLIS, D. (1994b) 'Care management', in N. Malin (ed.), *Implementing Community Care*, Buckingham: Open University Press

CHAPMAN, M. and MURIE, A. (1996) 'Housing and the European Union', *Housing Studies*, **11** (2), 307–18

CHAPMAN, T., GOODWIN, S. and HENNELLY, R. (1991) 'A new deal for the mentally ill: progress or propaganda?', *Critical Social Policy*, **32**, 5–20

CHAUDHARY, V. (1996) '"Harmless" lover who admired mass killers', *Guardian*, 10 December

CLAPHAM, D., KEMP, P., and SMITH, S. J. (1990) *Housing And Social Policy*, London: Macmillan

CLARKE, J. (1996) 'After social work?', in N. Parton (ed.), *Social Theory, Social Change and Social Work*, London: Routledge

CLARKE, J., COCHRANE, A. and MCLAUGHLIN, E. (1994) *Managing Social Policy*, London: Sage

CLARKE, J. and LANGAN, M. (1993) 'Restructuring welfare: the British welfare regime in the 1980s', in A. Cochrane and J. Clarke (eds), *Comparing Welfare States: Britain in international context*, London: Sage

CLARKE, J. and NEWMAN, J. (1997) *The Managerial State: Power, politics and ideology in the remaking of social welfare*, London: Sage

COCHRANE, A. (1993) 'Challenges from the centre', in J. Clarke (ed.), *A Crisis in Care?: Challenges to social work*, London: Sage

COCHRANE, A. (1994) 'Restructuring the local welfare state', in R. Burrows and B. Loader (eds), *Towards a Post-Fordist Welfare State*, London: Routledge

COHEN, A. (1985) *The Symbolic Construction of Community*, London: Tavistock

COLE, I. and FURBEY, R. (1994) *The Eclipse of Council Housing*, London: Routledge

COOKE, P. (ed.) (1989) *Localities*, London: Unwin Hyman

COOKE, P. (1990) *Back To The Future: Modernity, postmodernity and locality*, London: Unwin Hyman

COOPER, C. (1996) 'Lack of resources no excuse for no service', *Community Care*, 11–17 July, 9

COOPER, J. and VERNON, S. (1996) *Disability and the Law*, London: Jessica Kingsley

COPE, R. (1989) 'The compulsory detention of Afro-Caribbeans under the Mental Health Act', *New Community*, **15** (3), 346–56

CORNWELL, J. (1984) *Hard-earned Lives: Accounts of health and illness from East London*, London: Tavistock

CORNWELL, N. (1992) 'Assessment and accountability in community care', *Critical Social Policy*, **36**, 40–52

COWEN, H. (1994) *The Human Nature Debate: Social theory, social policy and the caring professions*, London: Pluto

CRAIG, G. (1996) '"Race", social security and poverty', paper delivered at Conference on Racism and Welfare, University of Central Lancashire, Preston, April

CRAIG, G. and RAI, D. K. (1996) 'Social security, community care and "race": the marginal dimension', in W. I. Ahmad and K. Atkin (eds), *'Race' and Community Care*, Buckingham: Open University Press

CROCKETT, N. and SPICKER, P. (1994) *Discharged: Homelessness Among Psychiatric Patients In Scotland: A study of the housing experience of discharged psychiatric patients and the role of care in the community*, Edinburgh: Shelter

CROFT, S. and BERESFORD, P. (1992) 'The politics of participation', *Critical Social Policy*, **35**, 20–44

CROW, G. and ALLAN, G. (1994) *Community Life: An introduction to local social relations*, Hemel Hempstead: Harvester Wheatsheaf

CURTIS, Z. (1995) 'Gaining confidence – speaking out', in R. Jack (ed.), *Empowerment in Community Care*, London: Chapman & Hall

DALLEY, G. (1988) *Ideologies of Caring: Rethinking community and collectivism*, London: Macmillan

DALLEY, G. (1996) *Ideologies of Caring: Rethinking community and collectivism*, 2nd edn, London: Macmillan

DALLEY, G. (1993) 'Professional ideology or organisational tribalism? The Health Service–social work divide?', in J. Walmsley, J. Reynolds, P. Shakespeare and R. Woolfe (eds), *Health, Welfare and Practice: Reflecting on roles and relationships*, London: Sage

DALY, G. B. J. (1996) 'Public accountability in today's health service', in H. Davis (ed.), *Quangos and Local Government: A changing world*, London: Cass

DANGERFIELD, R. (1936) *The Strange Death of Liberal England*, London: Serif

DAUNT, P. (1991) *Meeting Disability: A European response*, London: Cassell

DAVIES, B. P. and CHALLIS, D. J. (1986) *Matching Resources to Needs in Community Care*, Aldershot: Gower

DAVIS, A. (1991) 'Users' perspectives', in S. Ramon with M. G. Giannichedda (eds), *Psychiatry In Transition: The British and Italian experiences*, London: Pluto

DAVIS, K. (1993) 'On the movement', in J. Swain, V. Finklestein, S. French and M. Oliver (eds), *Disabling Barriers – Enabling Environments*, London: Sage

DAVIS, K. (1996) 'Disability and legislation: rights and equality' in G. Hales (ed.), *Beyond Disability: Towards an enabling society*, London: Sage

DAVIS, L. J. (1995) *Enforcing Normalcy: Disability, deafness and the body*, London: Verso

DAWSON, SIR A. (1994) *Homelessness and Ill Health*, report of Working Party on Homelessness and Ill Health, London: Royal College of Physicians

DEAKIN, N. (1994) *The Politics of Welfare: Continuities and change*, Hemel Hempstead: Harvester Wheatsheaf

DENNIS, N., HENRIQUES, F. and SLAUGHTER, C. (1969) *Coal Is Our Life: An analysis of a Yorkshire mining community*, London: Tavistock

DEPARTMENT OF HEALTH (1989) *Caring For People*, London: HMSO

DEPARTMENT OF HEALTH (1994) *A Framework for Community Care Charters in England*, London: HMSO

DEPARTMENT OF HEALTH (1995) *NHS Responsibilities for Meeting Continuing Health Care Needs*, London: HMSO, HSG (95) 8, LAC (95) 5

DHILLON-KASHYOP, P. (1994) 'Black women and housing', in R. Gilroy and R. Woods (eds), *Housing Women*, London: Routledge

DOBSON, F. (1996) 'Risks and rights', *Community Care*, 15–21 February

DOLING, J. (1993) 'Encouraging home ownership', in C. Jones (ed.), *New Perspectives on the Welfare State In Europe*, London: Routledge

DOMINELLI, L. (1991) *Women Across Continents: Feminist comparative social policy*, Hemel Hempstead: Prentice Hall/Harvester Wheatsheaf

DOMINELLI, L. (1996) 'Deprofessionalising social work: anti-oppressive practice, competence and postmodernism', *British Journal of Social Work*, **26**, 153–75

DOMINELLI, L. and HOOGVELT, A. (1996) 'Globalisation and the techno-cratization of social work', *Critical Social Policy*, **47**, 45–62

DOUGLAS, A. and GILROY, R. (1994) 'Young women and homelessness', in R. Gilroy and R. Woods (eds), *Housing Women*, London: Routledge

DOYAL, L. (1995) *What Makes Women Sick: Gender and the political economy of health*, London: Macmillan

DOYAL, L. and GOUGH, I. (1984) 'A theory of human need', *Critical Social Policy*, **10**, 6–38

DOYAL, L. and GOUGH, I. (1991) *A Theory of Human Need*, London: Macmillan

DOYLE, B. (1995) *Disability, Discrimination and Equal Opportunities: A comparative study of the employment rights of disabled persons*, London: Mansell

DRAKE, R. (1996) 'A critique of the role of the traditional charities', in L. Barton (ed.), *Disability and Society: Emerging issues and insights*, London: Longman

DROVER, G. and KERANS, P. (eds) (1993) *New Approaches To Welfare Theory*, Aldershot: Edward Elgar

EAGLETON, T. (1991) *Ideology: An introduction*, London: Verso

ELKIND, A. *et al.* (1995) 'Pass notes', *Health Service Journal*, 4 May, 30–1

ELSHTAIN, J. B. (1993) *Public Man, Private Woman: Women in social and political thought*, 2nd edn, Princeton, NJ: Princeton University Press

EMERSON, E. (1992) 'What is normalisation?', in H. Brown and H. Smith (eds), *Normalisation: A reader for the nineties*, London: Routledge

ESPING-ANDERSON, G. (1990) *The Three Worlds of Welfare Capitalism*, Cambridge: Polity

ESPING-ANDERSEN, G. (ed.) (1996) 'Welfare states without work: the impasse of labour shedding and familialism in continental European social policy', in id. (ed.), *Welfare States in Transition: National adaptations in global economies*, London: Sage

ETHERINGTON, S. (1996) 'To the millennium: the changing pattern of voluntary organisations', in C. Hanvey and T. Philpot (eds), *Sweet Charity: The role and workings of voluntary organisations*, London: Routledge

ETZIONI, A. (1993) *The Spirit of Community: Rights, responsibilities and the communitarian agenda*, London: Fontana

EVANDROU, M., FALKINGHAM, J. and GLENNERSTER, H. (1990) 'The personal social services: "everyone's poor relation but nobody's baby"', in J. Hills (ed.), *The State of Welfare*, Oxford: Clarendon Press

FARNHAM, D. and HORTON, S. (1993) 'Managing the new public services', in id. (eds), *Managing the New Public Services*, London: Macmillan

FARNHAM, D. and HORTON, S. (1996) 'Managing the new public services', in id. (eds), *Managing the New Public Services*, 2nd edn, London: Macmillan

FAWCETT, B. and FEATHERSTONE, B. (1996) '"Carers" and "caring": new thoughts on old questions' in B. Humphreys (ed.), *Critical Perspectives On Empowerment*, Birmingham: Venture Press

FELCE, D., BEYER, S. and TODD, S. (1995) 'A strategy for all seasons', *Community Care*, 3–9 August, 22–3

FENNELL, G., PHILLIPSON, C. and EVERS, H. (1988) *The Sociology of Old Age*, Buckingham: Open University Press

FERNANDO, S. (1991) *Mental Health, Race and Culture*, London: Macmillan/MIND

FIEDLER, B. (1991) *Tracking Success: Testing services for people with severe physical and sensory disabilities*, Project Paper no. 2, Living Options in Practice, London: King's Fund Centre

FINCH, J. (1984) 'Community care: developing non-sexist alternatives', *Critical Social Policy* (9), 6–18

FINCH, J. (1989) *Family Obligations and Social Change*, Cambridge: Polity

FLYNN, N. (1996) 'A mixed blessing? How the contract culture works', in C. Hanvey and T. Philpott (eds), *Sweet Charity: The role and workings of voluntary organisations*, London: Routledge

FLYNN, R., WILLIAMS, G. and PICKARD, S. (1996) *Markets and Networks: Contracting in community health services*, Buckingham: Open University Press

FORD, S. (1996) 'Learning difficulties', in G. Hales (ed.), *Beyond Disability: Towards an enabling society*, London: Sage

FORREST, R. and MURIE, A. (1991) *Selling The Welfare State*, London: Routledge

FOUCAULT, M. (1961) *Madness and Civilisation*, Harmondsworth: Penguin

FOUCAULT, M. (1973) *Birth of the Clinic*, Harmondsworth: Penguin

FRANCIS, J. (1996a) 'Fight on all sides', *Community Care*, 29 August–4 September, 12–3

FRANCIS, J. (1996b) 'Then and now: 25 years of social work', *Community Care*, 25 April–1 May, 20–21, special supplement

FRANCIS, J. (1996c) 'A brave new world', *Community Care*, 11–17 July, 18–19

FRANKENBERG, R. (1969) *Communities in Britain: Social life in town and country*, Harmondsworth: Penguin

FRASER, C. (1996) 'Just a housing problem?', *Roof*, November/December

FRASER, D. (1973) *The Evolution of the British Welfare State*, London: Macmillan

FRASER, D. (1984) *The Evolution of the British Welfare State*, 2nd edn, London: Macmillan

FRASER, N. and GORDON, L. (1994) 'Civil citizenship against social citizenship? On the ideology of contract versus charity', in B. van Steenbergen (ed.), *The Condition of Citizenship*, London: Sage

FRIEDMAN, M. (1992) 'Feminism and modern friendship: dislocating the community', in S. Avineri and A. de-Shalit (eds), *Communitarianism and Individualism*, Oxford: Oxford University Press

FRIEDMAN, M. with FRIEDMAN, R. (1962) *Capitalism and Freedom*, Chicago: Chicago University Press

FRIEDSON, E. (1970) *The Profession of Medicine*, New York: Harper & Row

GAMARNIKOW, E., MORGAN, D., PURVIS, J. and TAYLORSON, D. (eds) (1983) *The Public and the Private*, London: Heinemann

GANDHI, P. (1996) ' When I'm sixty-four: listening to what elderly people from ethnic minorities need', *Professional Social Work*, February, 12–13

GEORGE, M. (1995a) 'Needs Must . . .', *Community Care*, 28 September–4 October, 25

GEORGE, M (1995b) 'Put to the test', *Community Care*, 23–29 March,18

GEORGE, M. (1995c) 'Broken promises', *Community Care*, 24–30 August, 16

GEORGE, M. (1996) 'Figure it out', *Community Care*, 1–7 August

GEORGE, V. and Miller, S. (1994) 'The Thatcherite attempt to square the circle', in V. George and S. Miller (eds), *Social Policy Towards 2000: Squaring the welfare circle*, London: Routledge

GEORGE, V. and TAYLOR-GOOBY, P. (eds) (1996) *European Welfare Policy: Squaring the welfare circle*, London: Macmillan

GEORGE, V. and WILDING, P. (1994) *Welfare and Ideology*, Hemel Hempstead: Harvester Wheatsheaf

GIBSON, D. (1996) 'Reforming aged care in Australia: change and consequence', *Journal of Social Policy*, **25** (2), 157–79

GIDDENS, A. (1982) *Profiles and Critiques in Social Theory*, London: Macmillan

GILBERT, B. B. (1970) *British Social Policy 1914–1939*, London: Batsford

GILLIGAN, C. (1982) *In a Different Voice: Psychological theory and women's development*, Cambridge, MA: Harvard University Press

GINN, J. and ARBER, S. (1994) 'Heading for hardship: how the British pension system has failed women', in S. Baldwin and J. Falkingham (eds), *Social Security and Social Change*, Hemel Hempstead: Harvester Wheatsheaf

GINSBURG, N. (1992) *Divisions of Welfare: A critical introduction to comparative social policy*, London: Sage

GINSBURG, N. (1993) 'Sweden: the social democratic case', in A. Cochrane and J. Clarke (eds), *Comparing Welfare States*, London: Sage

GIUDICE, G. D., PASCALE, E. and REALE, M. (1991) 'How can mental hospitals be phased out?', in S. Ramon with M. G. Giannichedda (eds) *Psychiatry In Transition: The British and Italian experiences*, London: Pluto

GLENDINNING, C. (1988) 'Dependency and interdependency: the incomes of informal carers and the impact of social security', in S. Baldwin, G. Parker and R. Walker (eds), *Social Security and Community Care*, Aldershot: Avebury/Gower

GLENDINNING, C. (1992) '"Community care": the financial consequences for women', in C. Glendinning and J. Millar (eds), *Women and Poverty in Britain: The 1990s*, Hemel Hempstead: Harvester Wheatsheaf

GLENDINNING, C. and MCLAUGHLIN, E. (1993) *Paying for Care: Lessons from Europe*, London: HMSO

GLENDINNING, C. and MILLAR, J. (1991) 'Poverty – the forgotten Englishwoman: Reconstructing research and policy on poverty', in M. Maclean and D. Groves (eds), *Women's Issues in Social Policy*, London: Routledge

GOFFMAN, E. (1961) *Asylums*, Harmondsworth: Penguin

GOMM, R. (1993) 'Issues of power in health and welfare', in J. Walmsley, J. Reynolds, P. Shakespeare, R. Woolfe (eds), *Health, Welfare and Practice: Reflecting on roles and relationships*, London: Sage

GOODING, C. (1994) *Disabling Laws, Enabling Acts*, London: Pluto

GOODWIN, S. (1990) *Community Care And The Future of Mental Health Service Provision*, Aldershot: Avebury

GOULD, A. (1996) 'Sweden: the last bastion of social democracy', in V. George and P. Taylor-Gooby (eds), *European Welfare Policy: Squaring the welfare circle*, London: Macmillan

GRAHAM, H. (1983) 'Caring: a labour of love', in J. Finch and D. Groves (eds), *A Labour of Love: Women, work and caring*, London: RKP

GRANT, L. (1995) 'Head above water', *Community Care*, 16–22 November, 26–27

GRAY, J. (1997) *Endgames: Questions in late modern political thought*, Cambridge: Polity

GREEN, J. and SALTMAN, B. (1997) 'Primary health care', in D. Skidmore (ed.), *Community Care: Initial training and beyond*, London: Arnold

GRIFFITHS, SIR R. (1988) *Community Care: Agenda for action*, London: HMSO

GRIMSLEY, M. and BHAT, A. (1988) 'Health', in A. Bhat, R. Carr-Hill and S. Ohri (eds), *Britain's Black Population: A new perspective*, Aldershot: Gower

GROVES, D. (1992) 'Occupational pension provision and women's poverty in old age', in C. Glendinning and J. Millar (eds), *Women and Poverty in Britain: The 1990s*, Hemel Hempstead: Harvester Wheatsheaf

GROVES, D. and FINCH, J. (1983) 'Natural selection: perspectives on entitlement to the invalid care allowance', in J. Finch and D. Groves (eds), *A Labour of Love: Women, work and caring*, London: RKP

GROVES, E. (1997) 'Adult care', in D. Skidmore (ed.), *Community Care: Initial training and beyond*, London: Arnold

HABERMAN, S. and SCHMOOL, M. (1995) 'Estimates of the British Jewish population 1984–88', *Journal of the Royal Statistical Society A*, **158** (3), 547–62

HACKLER, C. (1995) 'Health care reform in the United States', in D. Seedhouse (ed.), *Reforming Health Care: The philosophy and practice of international health reform*, Chichester: Wiley

HADLEY, R. and CLOUGH, R. (eds) (1996) *Care in Chaos: Frustration and challenge in community care*, London: Cassell

HAM, C. and HEWITT, P. (1995) 'Where's the cure?', *Guardian*, 20 September

HANCOCK, C. (1995) 'What is long-term care?', *Health Service Journal*, 5 January, 15

HANMER, J. and SAUNDERS, S. (1984) *Well-Founded Fear: A community study of violence to women*, London: Hutchinson

HANTRAIS, L. (1995) *Social Policy in the European Union*, London: Macmillan

HARDEMAN, W. (n.d.) 'Promotion of consumer control in Dutch health care and social services', in D. Brandon (ed.), *Money for Change*, Cambridge: Anglia Polytechnic University

HARLOE, M. (1994) 'Social housing past, present and future: Policy Review', *Housing Studies*, **9** (3), 407–16

HARLOE, M. (1995) *The People's Home: Social rented housing in Europe and America*, Oxford: Blackwell

HARLOE, M., PICKVANCE, C. and URRY, J. (eds) (1990) *Place, Policy and Politics*, London: Unwin Hyman

HARRIS, C. (1987) *Redundancy and Recession in South Wales*, Oxford: Blackwell

HARRISON, M. (1993) 'The black voluntary housing movement: pioneering pluralistic social policy in a difficult climate', *Critical Social Policy*, **39**, 21–35

HARRISON, M. (1995) *Housing, 'Race', Social Policy and Empowerment*, Aldershot: Avebury

HARRISON, M. (1996) 'Empowerment and black-led housing associations: a decade of housing corporation programme, 1985–1995', paper delivered at Conference on Racism and Welfare, University of Central Lancashire, Preston, April

HARRISON, S., HUNTER, D. J., MARNOCH, G. and POLLITT, C. (1992) *Just Managing: Power and culture in the National Health Service*, London: Macmillan

HARRISON, S., HUNTER, D. J. and POLLITT, C. (1990) *The Dynamics of British Health Policy*, London: Unwin Hyman

HARRISON, T. (1995) *Disability: Rights and wrongs*, London: Lion

HARVEY, D. (1989) *The Condition of Postmodernity*, Oxford: Blackwell

HAYEK, F. (1962) *The Road To Serfdom*, London: RKP

HELD, D. (1984) *Political Theory And The Modern State: Essays on state, power and democracy*, Cambridge: Polity

HEWITT, M. (1992) *Welfare, Ideology and Need: Developing perspectives on the welfare state*, Hemel Hempstead: Harvester Wheatsheaf

HILL, D. (1994) *Citizenship and Cities*, Hemel Hempstead: Prentice Hall/Harvester Wheatsheaf

HILL, M. (1996) *Social Policy: A comparative analysis*, Hemel Hempstead: Prentice Hall/HarvesterWheatsheaf

HIRST, P. (1994) *Associative Democracy*, Oxford: Polity

HODGES, K. (1996) 'Policing the parsonage', *Housing Today*, 17 October, 13

HOGGETT, P. (1994) 'The politics of the modernisation of the UK welfare state', in R. Burrows and B. Loader (eds), *Towards A Post-Fordist Welfare State*, London: Routledge

HOLLIDAY, I. (1992) *The NHS Transformed: A guide to the health reforms*, Manchester: Baseline Books

HOLLIDAY, I. (1996) *The NHS Transformed: A guide to the health reforms*, 2nd edn, Manchester: Baseline Books

HOYES, L. and LART, R. (1992) 'Taking care', *Community Care*, 20 October, 14–15

HOYES, L. and MEANS, R. (1991) *Implementing the White Paper on Community Care*, Studies in Decentralisation and Quasi-Markets no. 4, Bristol: School for Advanced Urban Studies, University of Bristol

HOYES, L. and MEANS, R. (1993a) 'Markets, contracts and social care services: prospects and problems', in J. Bornat *et al.* (eds), *Community Care: A reader*, London: Macmillan

HOYES, L. and MEANS, R. (1993b) 'Quasi-markets and the reform of community care', in J. Le Grand and W. Bartlett (eds), *Quasi-Markets and Social Policy*, Bristol: School For Advanced Urban Studies

HUDSON, B. (1995) 'Could do better', *Health Service Journal*, 30 November, 30–1

HUGHES, B. (1995) *Older People and Community Care: Critical theory and practice*, Buckingham: Open University Press

HUGHES, M. (1995) 'The prospect is old age penury', *Guardian*, 2 October

HUGMAN, R. (1994) *Ageing and the Care of Older People in Europe*, London: Macmillan

HUMPHREYS, B. (1996) 'Contradictions in the culture of empowerment', in id. (ed.), *Critical Perspectives On Empowerment*, Birmingham: Venture Press

HUNTER, D. (1994a) 'The impact of the NHS reforms on community care', in M. Titterton (ed.), *Caring for People in the Community*, London: Jessica Kingsley

HUNTER, D. (1994b) 'From joint planning to community care planning: some lessons', in R. Davidson and S. Hunter (eds), *Community Care In Practice*, London: Batsford

HUSBAND, C. (1996) 'Defining and containing diversity: community, ethnicity and citizenship', in W. I. Ahmad and K. Atkin (eds), *'Race' and Community Care*, Buckingham: Open University Press

ITZEN, C. (1986) 'Ageism awareness training: a model for group work', in C. Phillipson, M. Bernard and P. Steang (eds), *Dependency and Inter-dependency in Old Age: Theoretical perspectives and policy alternatives*, London: Croom Helm

JACKSON, B. (1968) *Working Class Community: Some general notions raised by a series of studies in northern England*, London: RKP

JAMES, A. (1992) 'Quality and its social construction by managers in care service organisations', in D. Kelly and B. Warr (eds), *Quality Counts: Achieving quality in social care services*, London: Whiting & Birch

JAMES, A. (1994) *Managing to Care*, London: Longman

JARY, D. and JARY, J. (1995) *Dictionary of Sociology*, Glasgow: HarperCollins

JERROME, D. (1993) 'Intimate relationships', in J. Bond, P. Coleman and S. Peace (eds), *Ageing and Society: An introduction to social gerontology*, London: Sage

JESSOP, B. (1994) 'The transition to post-Fordism and the Schumpeterian workfare state', in R. Burrows and B. Loader (eds), *Towards A Post-Fordist Welfare State?*, London: Routledge

JEWISH COMMUNITY CARE FORUM OF GREATER MANCHESTER (1993) *Community Care in the Jewish Community of Greater Manchester and Cheshire*, First plan, Manchester: JCCF

JEWISH COMMUNITY CARE FORUM OF GREATER MANCHESTER (1995) *Community Care in the Jewish Community of Greater Manchester and Cheshire*, Second plan, Manchester: JCCF

JOHNSON, N. (1990) *Reconstructing the Welfare State: A decade of change, 1980–1990*, Hemel Hempstead: Harvester Wheatsheaf

JOHNSON, P. (1989) 'The structural dependency of the elderly: a critical note', in M. Jeffreys (ed.), *Growing Old in the Twentieth Century*, London: Routledge

JONES, C. (1996) 'Anti-intellectualism and the peculiarities of British social work education', in N. Parton (ed.), *Social Theory, Social Change And Social Work*, London: Routledge

JONES, D., LESTER, C. and WEST, R. (1993) 'Monitoring changes in health services for older people', in R. Robinson and J. Le Grand (eds), *Evaluating the NHS Reforms*, London: King's Fund

JONES, K. (1989) 'Community care: old problems and new answers', in P. Carter, T. Jeffs and M. Smith (eds), *Social Work and Social Welfare Year Book 1*, Milton Keynes: Open University Press

JONES, K. (1994) *The Making of Social Policy in Britain 1830–1990*, 2nd edn, London: Athlone Press

JONES, K. with BROWN, J., CUNNINGHAM, W. J., ROBERTS, J. and WILLIAMS, P. (1975) *Opening The Door: A study of new policies for the mentally handicapped*, London: RKP

JONES, S. (1993) *The Language of the Genes*, London: Flamingo

KEITH, L. (1996) 'Encounters with strangers: the public's responses to disabled women and how this affects our sense of self', in J. Morris (ed.), *Encounters with Strangers: Feminism and disability*, London: The Women's Press

KENT, I. (1996) 'Reporting back', *Community Care*, 22–28 February

KINGDOM, E. (1996) 'Gender and citizenship rights', in J. Demaine and H. Entwistle (eds), *Beyond Communitarianism: Citizenship, politics and education*, London: Macmillan

KLEIN, R. (1995) *The New Politics of the NHS*, 3rd edn, Harlow: Longman

KNOWLES, C. (1991) 'Afro-Caribbeans and schizophrenia', *Journal of Social Policy*, **20** (2), 173–90

KOHLER, M. (1996) 'How will we pay for her?', *Guardian*, 18 September, 7

KPMG Peat Marwick (1994) *Delivering the NHS Community Care Agenda*, London: NHS Executive

LAING, R. D. (1959) *The Divided Self*, London: Tavistock

LAND, H. (1978) 'Who cares for the family?', *Journal of Social Policy*, **7** (3), 257–84

LASH, S. and URRY, J. (1987) *The End of Organised Capitalism*, Cambridge: Polity

LASLETT, P. (1996) *A Fresh Map of Life: The emergence of the third age*, 2nd edn, London: Weidenfeld & Nicolson

LAVALETTE, M. and PRATT, A. (eds) (1997) *Social Policy: A conceptual and theoretical introduction*, London: Sage

LAW, I. (1996) *Racism, Ethnicity And Social Policy*, Hemel Hempstead: Prentice Hall/Harvester Wheatsheaf

LAWSON, R. (1993) 'The new technology of management in the personal social services', in P. Taylor-Gooby and R. Lawson (eds), *Markets and Managers: New issues in the delivery of welfare*, Buckingham: Open University Press

LEACH, B. (1996) 'Disabled people and the equal opportunities movement', in G. Hales (ed.), *Beyond Disability: Towards an enabling society*, London: Sage

LEE, P. and RABAN, C. (1988) *Welfare Theory and Social Policy*, London: Sage

LE GRAND, J. (1990) *Quasi-Markets and Social Policy*, Bristol: School For Advanced Urban Studies

LE GRAND, J. and BARTLETT, W. (eds) (1993) *Quasi-Markets and Social Policy*, London: Macmillan

LEWIS, J., BERNSTOCK, P. and BOVELL, V. (1995) 'The community care changes: unresolved tensions in policy and issues in implementation', *Journal of Social Policy*, **24** (1), January, 73–94

LEWIS, J. and GLENNERSTER, H. (1996) *Implementing The New Community Care*, Buckingham: Open University Press

LEWIS, J. and MEREDITH, B. (1988) *Daughters Who Care: Daughters caring for mothers at home*, London: RKP

LINDOW, V. (1995) 'Power and rights: the psychiatric system survivor movement', in R. Jack (ed.), *Empowerment in Community Care*, London: Chapman & Hall

LIPIETZ, A. (1988) 'Accumulation, crises and the ways out: some methodological reflections on the concept of "regulation"', *International Journal of Political Economy*, **18**, 10–43

LISTER, R. (1996) 'Citizenship, welfare rights and local government' in J. Demaine and H. Entwistle (eds), *Beyond Communitarianism: Citizenship, politics and education*, London: Macmillan

LITTLEWOOD, R. and LIPSEDGE, M. (1989) *Aliens and Alienists: Ethnic minorities and psychiatry*, 2nd edn, London: Routledge

LOADER, B. and BURROWS, R. (1994) 'Towards a post-Fordist welfare state? The restructuring of Britain, social policy and the future of welfare', in R. Burrows and B. Loader (eds), *Towards A Post-Fordist Welfare State?*, London: Routledge

LOCKWOOD, J. (1996) 'Mental health and young homeless link', *Housing Today*, 21 November

LODZIAK, C. (1995) *Manipulating Needs: Capitalism and culture*, London: Pluto

LONSDALE, S. (1990) *Women and Disability: The experience of physical disability among women*, Basingstoke: Macmillan

LONSDALE, S. and SEDDON, J. (1994) 'The growth of disability benefits: an international comparison', in S. Baldwin and J. Falkingham (eds), *Social Security and Social Change: New challenges to the Beveridge model*, Hemel Hempstead: Harvester Wheatsheaf

LORENZ, W. (1994) *Social Work in a Changing Europe*, London: Routledge

LOWE, R. (1993) *The Welfare State in Britain since 1945*, London: Macmillan

LOWRY, S. (1991) *Housing And Health*, London: BMJ

LUND, B. (1996) *Housing Problems and Housing Policy*, London: Longman

LUTHRA, M. (1997) *Britain's Black Population: Social Change, Public Policy and Agenda*, Aldershot: Arena/Ashgate

MCCABE, D. (1996) 'No place like home', *Community Care*, 22–28 August, 27

MACDONALD, K. M. (1995) *The Sociology of the Professions*, London: Sage

MCEWEN, E. (ed.) (1990) *Age – the Unrecognised Discrimination: Views to provoke a debate*, London: Age Concern England

MCGARVEY, N. and MIDWINTER, A. (1996) 'Reshaping social work authorities in Scotland', *British Journal of Social Work*, **26**, 201–21

MCGRATH, M. and HUMPHREYS, S. (1990) 'CMHTs at work: the Welsh experience', in S. Brown and G. Wistow (eds), *The Roles and Tasks of Community Mental Handicap Teams*, Aldershot: Avebury

MACINTYRE, A. (1985) *After Virtue: A study in moral theory*, 2nd edn, London: Duckworth

MACLEAN, M. and GROVES, D. (eds) (1991) *Women's Issues in Social Policy*, London: Routledge

MCNALLY, S. and ROSE, J. (1994) 'Day services', in N. Malin (ed.), *Implementing Community Care*, Buckingham: Open University Press

MALIN, N. (1994) 'Development of community care', in id. (ed.) *Implementing Community Care*: Buckingham: Open University Press

MALPASS, P. (1992) 'Housing policy and the disabling of local authorities', in J. Birchall (ed.), *Housing Policy in the 1990s*, London: Routledge

MAMA, A. (1992) 'Black women and the British state: race, class and gender analysis for the 1990s', in P. Braham, A. Rattansi and R. Skellington (eds), *Racism and Antiracism: Inequalities, opportunities and policies*, London: Sage

MANTHORPE, J. (1994) 'The family and informal care', in N. Malin (ed.), *Implementing Community Care*, Buckingham: Open University Press

MARSHALL, T. H. (1950) *Citizenship and Social Class*, London: Pluto

MASSEY, D. (1984) *The Spatial Divisions of Labour*, London: Macmillan

MASSEY, D. (1995) *The Spatial Divisions of Labour*, 2nd edn, London: Macmillan

MEANS, R. and LART, R. (1994) 'User empowerment, older people and the UK reform of community care', in R. Smith and J. Raistrick (eds), *Policy and Change*, Bristol: School For Advanced Urban Studies, University of Bristol

MEANS, R. and SMITH, R. (1994) *Community Care*, London: Macmillan

MEREDITH, B. (1995) *The Community Care Handbook*, 2nd edn, London: Age Concern England

MIDWINTER, E. (1994) *The Development of Social Welfare In Britain*, Buckingham : Open University Press

MISHRA, R. (1990) *The Welfare State in Capitalist Society: Policies of retrenchment and maintenance in Europe, North America and Australia*, Hemel Hempstead: Harvester Wheatsheaf

MODOOD, T., BERTHOUD, R., LAKEY, J., NAZROO, J., SMITH, P., VIRDEE, S. and BEISHON, S. (1997) *Ethnic Minorities in Britain: Diversity and disadvantage*, the Fourth National Survey of Ethnic Minorities, London: Policy Studies Institute

MOHAN. J. (1995) *A National Health Service? The Restructuring of Health Care in Britain since 1979*, London: Macmillan

MOORE, W. (1996) 'Proof has a price', *Guardian*, 6 December

MORRIS, J. (1991) *Pride Against Prejudice: Transforming attitudes to disability*, London: Women's Press

MORRIS, J. (1993) *Independent Lives: Community care and disabled people*, London: Macmillan

MORRIS, J. and KEITH, L. (1995) 'Easy targets: a disability rights perspective on the "children as carers" debate', *Critical Social Policy*, **44/45**, 36–57

MORRIS, L. and IRWIN, S. (1992) 'Unemployment and informal support: dependency, exclusion, or participation?', *Work, Employment and Society*, **6** (2), 185–207

MORRISON, E. and FINKLESTEIN, V. (1993) 'Broken arts and cultural repair: the role of culture in the empowerment of disabled people', in J. Swain, V. Finklestein, S. French and M. Oliver (eds), *Disabling Barriers – Enabling Environments*, London: Sage

MUIJEN, M. (1996) 'Mind maze', *Community Care*, 7–13 March

MULGAN, G. (ed.) (1997) *Life After Politics: New thinking for the twentieth century*, London: Fontana

MURPHY, E. (1991) *After The Asylums: Community care for people with mental illness*, London: Faber

NAVARRO, N. (1994) *The Politics of Health Policy: The US reforms, 1980–1994*, Oxford: Blackwell

NICHOLLS, V. (1997) 'Contracting and the voluntary sector: a critique of the impact of markets on Mind organizations', *Critical Social Policy*, **51**, May, 101–14

NIXON, J. (1993) 'Implementation in the hands of senior managers: community care in Britain', in M. Hill (ed.), *New Agendas in the Study of the Policy Process*, Hemel Hempstead: Prentice Hall/Harvester Wheatsheaf

NOCON, A. and QURESHI, H. (1996) *Outcomes of Community Care for Users and Carers*, Buckingham: Open University Press

NORMAN, A. (1985) *Triple Jeopardy: Growing old in a second homeland*, London: Centre For Policy on Ageing

NOZICK, R. (1974) *Anarchy, State and Utopia*, New York: Basic Books

OFFICE OF POPULATION CENSUS STATISTICS (1989) *General Household Survey 1986*, London: HMSO

OGG, J. and MUNN-GIDDINGS, C. (1993) 'Researching elder abuse', *Ageing and Society*, **13**, 389–413

O'KELL, S. (1996) 'Short changed', *Community Care*, 18–24 April, 26–7

OKIN, S. M. (1980) *Women in Western Thought*, London: Virago

OLIVER, D. and HEATER, D. (1994) *The Foundation of Citizenship*, Hemel Hempstead: Harvester Wheatsheaf

OLIVER, J. (1988) 'Social security and physical disability: a hidden issue', in S. Baldwin, G. Parker and R. Walker (eds), *Social Security and Community Care*, Aldershot: Avebury

OLIVER, M. (1990) *The Politics of Disablement*, London: Macmillan

OLIVER, M. (1996) *Understanding Disability*, London: Macmillan

OLIVER, M. and BARNES, C. (1993) 'Discrimination, disability and welfare: from needs to rights', in J. Swain, V. Finklestein, S. French and M. Oliver (eds), *Disabling Barriers – Enabling Environments*, London: Sage

OPPENHEIM, C. and HARKER, L. (1996) *Poverty: The facts*, 3rd edn, London: CPAG

O'SULLIVAN, N. (1993) 'Conservatism', in R. Eatwell and A. Wright (eds), *Contemporary Political Ideologies*, London: Pinter

OWEN, D. (1995) 'A quantitative profile of the African Caribbean community', in H. Goulbourne, H. Cowen, D. Owen with J. Blake, *The Needs of the African Caribbean Community in Coventry: A report*, Cheltenham: Centre for Policy and Health Research, Cheltenham & Gloucester CHE

PARKER, G. (1993) 'A four-way stretch? The politics of disability and caring', in J. Swain, V. Finklestein, S. French and M. Oliver (eds), *Disabling Barriers – Enabling Environments*, London: Sage

PASCALL, G. (1997) *Social Policy: A new feminist analysis*, 2nd edn, London: Routledge

PATEL, N. (1993) 'Healthy margins: black elders' care – models, policies and prospects', in W. I. Ahmad (ed.), *'Race' And Health In Contemporary Britain*, Buckingham: Open University Press

PAUL, S. (1996) 'Social workers take part in European fund contest', *Professional Social Work*, September, 8–9

PAYNE, M. (1995) *Social Work and Community Care*, London: Macmillan

PAYNE, S. (1991) *Women, Health and Poverty: An introduction*, Hemel Hempstead: Harvester Wheatsheaf

PETCH, A. (1994) '"The best move I've made": the role of housing for those with mental health problems', in M. Titterton (ed.), *Caring for People in the Community*, London: Jessica Kingsley

PETERS, M. and MARSHALL, J. (1996) *Individualism and Community: Education and social policy in the postmodern condition*, London: Falmer Press

PFEIFFER, D. (1994) 'Eugenics and disability discrimination', *Disability and Society*, **9** (4), 481–500

PHAROAH, C. and REDMOND, E. (1991), 'Care for ethnic elders', *Health Service Journal*, 16 May

PICKUP, l. (1988) 'Hard to get around: a study of women's travel mobility', in J. Little, L. Peake and P. Richardson (eds), *Women in Cities: Gender and the urban environment*, London: Macmillan

PICKVANCE, C. (1991) 'The difficulty of control and the ease of structural reform: British local government in the 1980s', in C. Pickvance and E. Preteceille (eds), *State Restructuring and Local Power: A comparative perspective*, Oxford: Blackwell

PIERSON, C. (1994) 'Continuity and discontinuity in the emergence of the "post-Fordist" welfare state', in R. Burrows and B. Loader (eds), *Towards a Post-Fordist Welfare State*, London: Routledge

PILCHER, J. (1995) *Age and Generation in Modern Britain*, Oxford: Oxford University Press

PILGRIM, D. (1993) 'Mental health services in the twenty-first century: the user–professional divide?', in J. Bornat *et al.* (eds), *Community Care : A reader*, London: Macmillan

PLANT, R. (1974) *Community and Ideology*, London: RKP

PLANT, R. (1988) *Citizenship, Rights and Socialism*, Fabian Society Pamphlet no. 531, London: Fabian Society

PLANT, R. (1991) *Modern Political Thought*, Oxford: Blackwell

PROFESSIONAL SOCIAL WORK (1996) 'Report of House of Commons Health Select Committee', *Professional Social Work*, September

QURESHI, H. (1996) 'Obligations and support within families', in A. Walker (ed.), *The New Generational Contract: Intergenerational relations, old age and welfare*, London: UCL Press

RACE, D. (1995) 'Classification of people with learning disabilities', in N. Malin (ed.), *Services for people with learning disabilities*, London: Routledge

RACK, P. (1982) *Race, Culture And Mental Disorder*, London: Tavistock

RAO, N. (1991) *From Providing To Enabling: Local authorities and community care planning*, York: Joseph Rowntree Foundation

RAWLS, J. (1974) *A Theory of Justice*, Oxford: Oxford University Press

READING, P. (1994) *Community Care and the Voluntary Sector*, Birmingham: Venture Press

REES, A. (1985) *T. H. Marshall's Social Policy*, 5th edn, London: Hutchinson

RENSHAW, J. (1994) 'Planning for community health care', in R. Davidson, and S. Hunter (eds), *Community Care In Practice*, London: Batsford

RENSHAW, J. (1995) 'Quality measurement in the all-Wales strategy', in D. Pilling and G. Watson (eds), *Evaluating Quality in Services for Disabled and Older People*, London: Jessica Kingsley

REULER, J. (1993) 'The American experience', in K. Fisher and J. Collins, (eds), *Health, Homelessness and Housing*, London: Routledge

RIMMER, L. (1983) 'The economics of work and caring', in J. Finch and V. Groves (eds), *A Labour of Love: Women, work and caring*, London: RKP

RITCHIE, P. (1994) 'The process of quality assurance', in R. Davidson and S. Hunter (eds), *Community Care in Practice*, London: Batsford

ROBERTS, H. (1982) 'Women, the "community" and the Family', in A. Walker (ed.), *Community Care: The family, the state and social policy*, London: Basil Blackwell and Martin Robertson

ROGERS, A. and PILGRIM, D. (1989) 'Citizenship and mental health', *Critical Social Policy*, **26**, 25–32

ROGERS, A. and PILGRIM, D. (1996) *Mental Health Policy In Britain: A critical introduction*, London: Macmillan

ROGERS, A., PILGRIM, D. and LACEY, R. (1993) *Experiencing Psychiatry: Users' views of services*, London: Macmillan

ROGERS, S. and BERENS, C. (1996) 'Homeless casualty crisis', *The Big Issue*, 16–29 December

ROSKILL, C. (1994) 'Echoes of the Holocaust', *Community Care*, 14 April, 25

ROSTRON, J. (1995) *Housing the Physically Disabled: An anthology and reader of practice and policy*, Aldershot: Arena

ROWE, A. (ed.) (1990) *Lifetime Homes: Flexible housing for successive generations*, London: Helen Hamlyn Foundation

Runnymede Commission on Anti-Semitism (1994) *A Very Light Sleeper: The persistence and dangers of anti-Semitism*, London: Runnymede Trust

RYAN, J. with THOMAS, F. (1987) *The Politics of Mental Handicap*, 2nd edn, London: Free Association Books

SAHLIN, I. (1995) 'Strategies for Exclusion from Social Housing', *Housing Studies*, **10** (3), 381–401

SALISBURY, B. (n.d.) 'Where do we go from here?', in B. Brandon (ed.), *Money For Change*, Cambridge: Anglia Polytechnic University

SAMPSON, C. and SOUTH, N. (1996) 'Introduction: social policy isn't what it used to be – the social construction of social policy in the 1980s and 1990s', in C. Sampson and N. South (eds), *The Social Construction of Social Policy: Methodologies, racism, citizenship and the environment*, London: Macmillan

SANDEL, M. (1982) *Liberalism and the Limits of Justice*, Cambridge: Cambridge University Press

SANDEL, M. (1992) 'The procedural republic and the unencumbered self', in S. Avineri and A. de-Shalit (eds), *Communitarianism And Individualism*, Oxford: Oxford University Press

SANDVIN, J. T. (1994) 'Reform or disassembling? Towards community services in Norway', *Care In Place*, **1** (1), March, 43–52

SASHIDHARAN, S. (1989) 'Schizophrenia or just black?', *Community Care*, **783**, 14–15

SASSOON, M. and LINDOW, V. (1995) 'Consulting and empowering Black mental health system users', in S. Fernando (ed.), *Mental Health in a Multi-ethnic Society*, London: Routledge

SCRUTTON, S. (1990) 'The foundation of age discrimination', in E. McEwen (ed.), *Age: The Unrecognised Discrimination: Views to provoke a debate*, London: Age Concern England

SCULL, D. (1977) *Decarceration: Community Treatment and the Deviant: A radical view*, Englewood Cliffs, NJ: Prentice-Hall

SEN, K. (1994) *Ageing: Debates on demographic transition and social policy*, London: Zed

SEXTY, C. (1990) *Women Losing Out: Access to housing in Britain today*, London: Shelter

SHAKESPEARE, T. (1993) 'Disabled people's self-organisation: a new social movement', *Disability, Handicap and Society*, **8** (3), 249–64

SHAPIRO, J. *et al.* (1996) 'Fluid Drives', *Health Service Journal*, 27 June, 28–31

SHONFIELD, A. (1969) *Modern Capitalism*, Oxford: Oxford University Press

SIIM, B. (1990) 'Women and the welfare state: between private and public dependence: a comparative approach to care work in Denmark and Britain', in C. Ungerson (ed.), *Gender and Caring*, Hemel Hempstead: Harvester Wheatsheaf

SIMIC, P. (1994) 'Moving out of hospital into the community', in M. Titterton (ed.), *Caring for People in the Community*, London: Jessica Kingsley

SKELLINGTON, R. with MORRIS, P. (1996) *'Race' In Britain Today*, 2nd edn, London: Sage

SKIDMORE, D. (1994) *The Ideology of Community Care*, London: Chapman & Hall

SLATER, P. (1995) 'From "elder protection" to "adult empowerment": critical reflections on a UK campaign', in R. Jack (ed.), *Empowerment in Community Care*, London: Chapman & Hall

SMITH, H. and BROWN, H. (1989) 'Whose community, whose care?', in A. Brechin and J. Walmsley (eds), *Making Connections: Reflecting on the lives and experiences of people with learning difficulties*, London: Hodder & Stoughton

SNELL, J. (1996) 'Fighting for survival', *Community Care*, 18–24 April, 14–15

SOCIAL SERVICES INSPECTORATE, DEPARTMENT OF HEALTH and GLOUCESTERSHIRE COUNTY COUNCIL SOCIAL SERVICES, GLOUCESTERSHIRE RACIAL EQUALITY COUNCIL (1991) *A Summary of Black Elders Living in the City of Gloucester*, Gloucester: Social Services Inspectorate *et al.*

SOLOMOS, J. and BACK, L. (1996) *Racism and Society*, London: Macmillan

SPICKER, P. (1993) *Housing And Community Care In Scotland*, Edinburgh: Shelter/Scottish Campaign For Homeless People

STEVENSON, J. (1984) *British Society: 1914–45*, The Pelican Social History of Britain, Harmondsworth: Penguin

STRONG, S. (1996) 'Recording contract', *Community Care*, 18–24 July, 25

STUART, O. (1992) 'Race and disability: what type of double disadvantage?', *Disability, Handicap and Society*, **7** (2), 177–88

STUART, O. (1996) ' "Yes, we mean black disabled people too": thoughts on community care and disabled people from blacks and minority ethnic communities', in W. I. Ahmad and K. Atkin (eds), *'Race' and Community Care*, Buckingham: Open University Press

STURGES, P. J. (1996) 'Care management practice: lessons from the USA', in C. Clark and I. Lapsley (eds), *Planning and Costing Community Care*, Research Highlights in Social Work no. 27, London: Jessica Kingsley

SULLIVAN, M. (1994) *Modern Social Policy*, Hemel Hempstead: Harvester Wheatsheaf

SULLIVAN, M. (1996) *The Development of the British Welfare State*, Hemel Hempstead: Prentice Hall/Harvester Wheatsheaf

SWITHIBANK, A. (1996) 'The European Union and social care', in B. Munday and P. Ely (eds), *Social Care in Europe*, Hemel Hempstead: Prentice Hall/Harvester Wheatsheaf

SZASZ, T. (1961) *The Myth of Mental Illness: A critical assessment of the Freudian approach*, London: Secker & Warburg

TAWNEY, R. H. (1931) *Equality*, London: Unwin Books

TAYLOR, C. (1989) *Sources of the Self*, Cambridge: Cambridge University Press

TAYLOR, D. (1989) 'Citizenship and social power', *Critical Social Policy*, **26**, 19–31

TAYLOR, M., LANGAN, J. and HOGGETT, P. (1995) *Encouraging Diversity: Voluntary and private organisations in community care*, Aldershot: Arena

TAYLOR-GOOBY, P. (1995) 'Comfortable, marginal and excluded: who should pay higher taxes for a better welfare state?', in R. Jowell, J. Curtice, A. Park, A. Brook, D. Ahrendt with K. Thomson (eds), *British Social Attitudes: The 12th report*, Social and Community Planning Research, Aldershot: Dartmouth

TESTER, S. (1996a) *Community Care For Older People: A comparative perspective*, London: Macmillan

TESTER, S. (1996b) 'Women and community care', in C. Hallett (ed.), *Women and Social Policy: An introduction*, Hemel Hempstead: Prentice Hall/Harvester Wheatsheaf

THAIN, J. (1995) 'Not too "grey" power', in R. Jack (ed.), *Empowerment in Community Care*, London: Chapman & Hall

THANE, P. (1996) *Foundations of the Welfare State*, 2nd edn, London: Longman

TIMMINS, N. (1996) *The Five Giants: A biography of the welfare state*, London: Fontana

TIMMS, P. (1993) 'Mental health and homelessness', in K. Fisher and J. Collins (eds), *Health, Homelessness and Housing*, London: Routledge

TINKER, A. (1992) *Elderly People in Modern Society*, London: Macmillan

TINKER, A. (1997) *Elderly People in Modern Society*, 2nd edn, London: Macmillan

TOMLINSON, D. (1996) 'The American, Flemish and British cases of asylum', in D. Tomlinson and J. Carrier (eds), *Asylum In The Community*, London: Routledge

TONNIES, F. (1955) *Community and Society* , tr. and ed. by C. P. Loomis, New York: Harper & Row

TOWNSEND, P. (1962) *The Last Refuge: A survey of residential institutions and homes for the aged in England and Wales*, London: RKP

TOWNSEND, P. (1963) *The Family Life of Old People*, Harmondsworth: Penguin

TOWNSEND, P. (1979) *Poverty in the United Kingdom: A survey of household resources and standards of living*, Harmondsworth: Penguin

TOWNSEND, P. (1981) 'The structured dependency of the elderly: a creation of social policy in the twentieth century', *Ageing and Society*, **1** (1), 5–28

TYNE, A. (1982) 'Community care and mentally handicapped people', in A. Walker (ed.), *Community Care: The family, the state and social policy*, Oxford: Basil Blackwell and Martin Robertson

UNGERSON, C. (1983a) 'Why do women care?', in J. Finch and V. Grove (eds), *Labour of Love: Women, work and caring*, London: RKP

UNGERSON, C. (1983b) 'Women and caring: skills, tasks and taboos', in E. Gamarnikow, D. Morgan, J. Purvis and D. Taylorson (eds), *The Public and the Private*, London: Heinemann

UNGERSON, C. and KEMBER, M. (1987) *Policy is Personal: Sex, gender and informal care*, London: Tavistock

UNGERSON, C. (ed.) (1997) *Women and Social Policy: A reader*, 2nd edn, London: Macmillan

VALIOS, N. (1996) 'Disaster time', *Community Care*,17–23 October, 12–13

WAERNESS, K. (1990) 'Informal and formal care in old age', in C. Ungerson (ed.) *Gender and Caring: Work and welfare in Britain and Scandinavia*, Hemel Hempstead: Harvester Wheatsheaf

WAGNER, DAME G. *et al.* (1996) *Building Expectations: Opportunities and services for people with a learning disability*, London: Mental Health Foundation

WALBY, S. and GREENWELL, J (1994) 'Managing the National Health Service', in J. Clarke, A. Cochrane and E. McLaughlin (eds), *Managing Social Policy*, London: Sage

WALKER, A. (ed.) (1982) *Community Care: The family, the state and social policy*, Oxford: Basil Blackwell and Martin Robertson

WALKER, A. (1990) 'Poverty and inequality in old age', in J. Bond and P. Coleman (eds), *Ageing in Society*, London: Sage

WALKER, A. (1992) 'The poor relation: poverty among older women', in C. Glendinning and J. Millar (eds), *Women and Poverty in Britain: The 1990s*, Hemel Hempstead: Harvester Wheatsheaf

WALKER, A. (1993) 'Community care policy: from consensus to conflict', in J. Bornat *et al.* (eds), *Community Care: A reader*, London: Macmillan

WALKER, R. and AHMAD, W. (1994) 'Windows of opportunity in rotting frames? Care providers' perspectives on community care and black communities', *Critical Social Policy*, **40**, 46–69

WALMSLEY, J. (1993) 'Contradictions in caring: reciprocity and inter-dependence', *Disability, Handicap and Society*, **8** (2), 129–41

WALZER, M. (1983) *Spheres of Justice: A defence of pluralism and equality*, Oxford: Blackwell

WARDE, A. (1994) 'Consumers, consumption and post-Fordism', in R. Burrows and B. Loader (eds), *Towards a Post-Fordist Welfare State*, London: Routledge

WATSON, S. with AUSTERBERRY, H. (1986) *Housing And Homelessness: A feminist perspective*, London: RKP

WATTERS, C. (1996) 'Representations and realities: black people, community care and mental illness', in W. I. Ahmad and K. Atkin (eds), *'Race' And Community Care*, Buckingham: Open University Press

WEAVER, M. (1996) 'Cut to the bone', *Housing Today*, **11**, 28 November

WEBER, M. (1946) *From Max Weber: Essays in sociology*, tr. and ed. H. Gerth and C. W. Mills, New York: Oxford University Press

WEBER, M. (1958) *The City*, tr. and ed. D. Martindale and G. Neuwith, New York: Free Press

WEIR, M. (1993) 'From equal opportunity to "the new social contract": race and the politics of the American "underclass"', in M. Cross and M. Keith (eds), *Racism, the City and the State*, London: Routledge

WELCH, C. (1996) 'Key issues in support', in G. Hales (ed.), *Beyond Disability: Towards an enabling society*, London: Sage

WETHERLY, P. (1996) 'Basic needs and social policies', *Critical Social Policy*, **46**, 45–65

WHITE, C. (1996) 'Structural damage', *Community Care*, 26 September–2 October

WHITELEY, P. (1996) 'Mental health discharge rules provoke furore', *Community Care*, 15–21 February

WHITELEY, P. and VALIOS, N. (1996) 'Commission defends diverse voluntary sector in England', *Community Care*, 11–17 July, 8–9

WHITTAKER, T. (1995) 'Gender and elder abuse', in S. Arber and J. Ginn (eds), *Connecting Gender and Ageing*, Buckingham: Open University Press

WILLIAMS, B. (1988) *Manchester Jewry: A pictorial history 1788–1988*, Manchester: Archive Publications

WILLIAMS, F. (1989) 'Mental handicap and oppression', in A. Brechin and J. Walmsley (eds), *Making Connections: Reflecting on the lives and experiences of people with learning difficulties*, London: Hodder & Stoughton

WILLIAMS, F. (1993) 'Women and community', in J. Bornat *et al.* (eds), *Community Care: A reader*, London: Macmillan

WILLIAMS, F. (1996) '"Race", welfare and community care: a historical perspective', in W. I. Ahmad and K. Atkin (eds), *'Race' And Community Care*, Buckingham: Open University Press

WILLIAMS, R. (1958) *Culture and Society*, Harmondsworth: Penguin

WILLIAMS, R. (1965) *The Long Revolution*, Harmondsworth: Penguin

WILLIAMS, R. (1983) *Keywords: A vocabulary of culture and society*, 2nd edn, London: Flamingo/Fontana

WILLMOTT, P. (ed.) (1986) *The Debate About Community*, London: PSI

WILLMOTT, P. and YOUNG, M. (1957) *Family and Kinship in East London*, London: RKP

WILSON, E. (1977) *Women and the Welfare State*, London: Tavistock

WILSON, E. (1991) *The Sphinx in the City: Urban life, the control of disorder*, London: Virago

WILSON, V. (1996) 'People with disabilities' in B. Munday and P. Ely (eds), *Social Care in Europe*, Hemel Hempstead: Prentice Hall/Harvester Wheatsheaf

WING, H. (1992) 'The role of inspection and evaluation in social care', in D. Kelly and B. Warr (eds), *Quality Counts: Achieving quality in social care services*, London: Whiting & Birch

WISTOW, G. (1994) 'Community care futures: inter-agency relationships – stability or continuing change', in M. Titterton (ed.), *Caring for People in the Community*, London: Jessica Kingsley

WISTOW, G. (1995) 'Coming apart at the seams', *Health Service Journal*, **2**, March, 24–5

WISTOW, G. and HARDY, B. (1994) 'Community care planning', in N. Malin (ed.) *Implementing Community Care*, Buckingham: Open University Press

WISTOW, G., HARDY, B., and ALLEN, C. (1994) *Social Care in a Mixed Economy*, Buckingham: Open University Press

WOLFENSBURGER, W. (1972) *The Principle of Normalisation in Human Services*, Toronto: National Institute on Mental Retardation

WRIGHT, A. (1993) 'Social democracy and democratic socialism', in R. Eatwell and A. Wright (eds), *Contemporary Political Ideologies*, London: Pinter

ZARB, G. (1993) 'The dual experience of ageing with a disability', in J. Swain, V. Finklestein, S. French and M. Oliver (eds), *Disabling Barriers–Enabling Environments*, London: Sage

ZARB, G. and OLIVER, M. (1992) *Ageing with a Disability: The dimensions of need*, London: Thames Polytechnic

INDEX

Abberley, P., 133
Abercrombie, N., 10
accountability, 20, 24, 57, 58, 90, 96,
    124, 193, 194, 198, 199, 201,
    203
advocacy and Citizen Advocacy
    Project, 158
ageism, 50, 114–16, 206,
    elder abuse, 115
    racism, discrimination and
        disablism, 114–15,
    sexism, 115
Ahmad, W. I., 91, 115, 181, 183, 191
Alaszewski, A., 78
Alber, J., 73, 104, 127
Alcock, P., 25, 89, 193
Alderman, G., 186, 191
Aldridge, J., 138
Allan, G., 4, 5, 170
Allen, D., 153
Allen, I., 124
Allsop, J., 54, 58, 59, 60, 67
Ambrose, P., 72
Anderson, B., 4
anti-Semitism, 188
Anttonen, A., 104
Arber, S., 114, 120, 121, 122, 129,
    165, 171, 172, 173, 174
Ashton, T., 72
Atkin, K., 79, 91, 183, 185, 191
Atkinson, D., 210

Audit Commission, 64, 67, 80, 97, 194
Austerberry, H., 152
Austin, R., 156

Back, L., 180
Bagguley, P., 11
Baldock, J., 168
Baldwin, S., 94, 121, 122, 165, 168,
    172, 175
Bannerman, L., 100
Barbalet, J., 193
Barham, P., 158
Barker, R., 16
Barnes, C., 21, 33, 39, 41, 131, 133,
    134, 135, 141
Barnes, M., 195, 198, 203
Bartlett, W., 56, 60
Barton, L., 141
Bean, P., 153
Beauchamp, D. E., 72
Beazley, M., 102
Begum, N., 99, 115
Begum, W., 174
Bell, C., 4
Bellamy, R., 27, 28
Bennet, G., 116
Benzeval, M., 7
Berens, C., 152
Beresford, P., 198
Berman, M., 12
Beuret, K., 170

Beveridge, William, 34, 35, 36, 37, 208
Bewley, C., 140
Bhat, A., 185
Biggs, S., 114
Blakemore, K., 113, 115, 129, 180, 181, 182, 184
Bland, R., 62, 98
Bond, J., 112
Boneham, M., 115, 129, 180, 181, 182, 184
Bornat, J., 5, 111
Borrie, G., 7, 199
Bowes, A., 191
Bradley, J., 103
Bradshaw, J., 6
Brandon, D., 161
Braybon, J., 142
Brenton, M., 32
Brindle, D., 60, 61, 142
Brooks, E. R., 162
Brown, G. W., 65, 152, 173
Brown, H., 133
Brown, J., 103
Brown, M., 131, 135
Bryan, B., 4
Bryson, L., 189
Bubeck, D., 177
Bulmer, M., 5, 8, 9
Burrows, R., 76
Butcher, H., 170
Butler, N., 114
Butt, J. 182, 183
Bytheway, W., 114

Cahill, M., 18
Cain, H., 4
Campbell, D., 156
care management and implementation, 97–100, 100–1
  Kent project, 97–8
Carers' (Recognition and Services) Act 1995, 80
'Caring For People' (1989), 61, 62–3, 68, 80, 81, 82–3, 97, 124, 153
Carlisle, D., 148
Carpenter, M., 67, 68, 90, 103
Carter, T., 125
Cashmore, E., 180

Cassam, E., 102
Caughey, J., 103
Cervi, B., 90, 120
Chadda, D., 64
Chadwick, A., 142
Challis, D., 97, 98, 100
Chapman, M., 160
Chapman, T., 68
Chaudhary, V., 156
Chronically Sick and Disabled Persons Act 1973, 140
citizenship and rights, 18, 24, 45, 58, 107, 115, 157, 158, 193–4
Citizen's Charter and consumerism, 57, 134, 195–6
citizenship and disability rights, 141, 142, 145, 146
civil rights and collective organisation, 140–2
Clapham, D., 139
Clarke, J., 16, 17, 85, 86, 102
Clough, R., 20, 103
Cochrane, A., 46, 84
Cohen, A., 5
Cole, I., 44, 151
collaboration, health–social care, 61–2, 63–4, 68, 70, 72–3, 205
  Denmark, France, Italy, Netherlands, USA, 73
  in community care plans, 96–7
  Spain, 105
community care and funding plans, 94–7
Community Health councils, 57
communitarianism and values, 199–202, 203, 208
  Etzioni's new communitarianism, 200–1, 218
contracts, culture, 12, 56, 58, 102, 185, 196, 200, 202, 205
  and social care market, 88–9
  and voluntary sector, 89–90, 91, 195
Cooke, P., 12, 84
Cooper, C., 95
Cooper, J., 132, 133, 135, 141, 145, 147
Cope, R., 71
Cornwell, J., 4

Cornwell, N., 99
Craig, G., 122, 123, 184
Crockett, N., 153
Croft, S., 198
Crow, G., 4, 5, 170
Curtis, Z., 125

Dalley, G., 8, 9, 18, 61, 165, 169, 173, 174, 177
Daly, G. B. J., 198, 199
Daly, Gerald., 163
Dangerfield, R., 32
Daunt, P., 144
Davies, B. P., 98
Davis, A., 157
Davis, K., 140, 141, 145, 146
Davis, L. J., 133, 137
Dawson, Sir A., 149, 150, 155
day care, 77–8
Deakin, N., 37, 43
dementia, 65
Dennis, N., 5
Dhillon-Kashyop, P., 152
disability, international policies, 142–6
disability, models of, 132–3, 142, 145, 146
    disability and disabled persons' movement, 140, 141, 145
    British Council of Organisations of Disabled People, 181
    National Disability Council, 142
    Denmark, Italy, Netherlands, 143
Disability Discrimination Act 1996, 142
disability benefits and financial difficulties, 135–6, 143
    Australia, Denmark, France, Germany, Sweden, USA, 143
Disabled Persons International, 144, 145
Disabled Persons (Services, Consultation and Representation) Act 1986, 140
disability rights and citizenship, 141, 142, 146, 147
    and community care legislation, 140

Gloucestershire CC judgment, 94–5
    and user involvement, 145–6
    Australia, Canada, European Union, Scandinavia, USA, 145
Dobson, F., 156
Doling, J., 160
domiciliary care, 78–9, 118
    Greece, Spain, Portugal, 126
Dominelli, L., 101, 102, 175
Douglas, A., 152
Doyal, Len, 6, 7
Doyal, Lesley, 173
Doyle, B., 145
Drake, R., 181, 195
Drover, G., 19

Eagleton, T., 14
elder abuse, 115–16
    Canada, USA, 116
Elkind, A., 64
Elshtain, J. B., 165, 167
Emerson, E., 136
empowerment, xv, 10, 18, 24, 99, 124–6, 130, 148, 157–9, 161–2, 197–9, 203, 209
    and minority ethnic groups, 91, 125
Enthoven, Alain, 52, 61, 72
Esping-Andersen, G., 126, 175
Etherington, S., 185
Etzioni, A., 200, 201, 203
European Community social policy, 1994, 144
European Convention for Protection of Human Rights, 145
European Union, 105, 107, 144, 145
Evandrou, M., 41

Fabianism, 16, 27–8
familialism, 9, 46, 168, 175, 176, 210
family and caring, 165–6
    African-Caribbean and Asian, 183–4
    Chinese, 185
    Jewish, 184–5
family and financial social policies, 175
    Denmark, Germany, Sweden, 175
Farnham, D., 16

Fawcett, B., 198
Featherstone, B., 198
Felce, D., 137
feminist perspectives of caring, debates, 173–5
Fennell, G., 115
Fernando, S., 71
Fiedler, B., 138
Finch, J., 113, 172, 173, 174
Finklestein, V., 133
Flynn, N., 88
Flynn, R., 88
Ford, S., 131, 132
Forrest, R., 44, 151
Foster, M., 116
Foucault, M., 66
Francis, J., 92, 103, 134
Frankenberg, R., 5
Fraser, C., 149
Fraser, D., 30, 32, 35, 37
Fraser, N., 196
Friedman, Marion, 201
Friedman, Milton, 15, 28, 43
Friedson, E., 51
Furbey, R., 44, 151

Galton, Francis, 33
Gamarnikow, E., 165
Gandhi, P., 125
George, M., 76, 94, 133, 136, 140
George, V., 34, 35, 43, 105, 107
Gibson, D., 126
Giddens, A., 194
Gilbert, B. B., 34
Gilligan, C., 167
Gilroy, R., 152
Ginn, J., 114, 120, 121, 122, 129, 165, 171, 172, 173, 174
Ginsburg, N., 72, 105, 126, 175, 189, 190
Giudice, G. D., 73
Glendenning, C., 122, 127, 140, 171
Glennerster, H., 61, 62, 63, 78, 79, 86, 88, 89, 90, 92, 94, 96, 100
global forces, and social services, 101–2, 103, 106
Goffman, E., 10, 30, 39, 66, 133, 173
Gomm, R., 197

Gooding, C., 141
Goodwin, S., 65, 66
Gordon, L., 196
Gostrick, C., 107
Gough, I., 6, 7
Gould, A., 105
GP fund-holding, 53, 54, 60, 63–5, 116, 205, 209
Graham, H., 165, 167
Grant, L., 136
Gray, J., 16
Green, J., 54
Greenwell, J., 55
Griffiths, Sir R., 44, 51–2, 80, 81, 82, 89, 97, 118, 153
Grimsley, M., 185
Groves, D., 18
Groves, D., 122, 172, 174
Groves, E., 53
Gupta, H., 102

Haberman, S., 178
Hackler, C., 72
Hadley, R., 20, 103
Ham, C., 59
Hancock, C., 123
Hanmer, J., 170
Hantrais, L., 105, 112, 144, 189
Hanvey, C., 107
Hardeman, W., 144
Hardy, B., 63, 86, 87, 96
Harker, L., 121, 122, 123, 135, 136
Harloe, M., 84,160
Harris, C., 11
Harris, T., 65, 152, 173
Harrison, M., 91
Harrison, S., 57, 58, 69
Harrison, T., 133
Harvey, D., 14, 84
Hayek, F., 15, 28, 43
health care reforms, 71–2
  Belgium, France, Germany, Ireland, Netherlands, New Zealand, Spain, UK, USA, 72
Heater, D., 193, 195, 196
Held, D., 194
Hewitt, M., 43
Hewitt, P., 59

Hill, D., 199
Hill, M., 18, 51, 59
Hirst, P., 202
Hodges, K., 155
Hoggett, P., 25, 89, 101, 197
Holliday, I., 54, 55, 58, 72
Holocaust, 188
homelessness and housing policies, 24,
     44, 68, 150–3, 156, 162
  and mental health, 148–50, 155,
     206–7
  and US McKinney Homeless
     Assistance Act 1987, 160–1
Hoogvelt, A., 101, 102
Horton, S., 16
housing associations, 139, 153, 154
Housing Corporation, 151
housing policies, 7, 19, 47, 134–5,
     146, 147, 150–2, 154, 170, 205
  grants, 138–9
  Housing Act 1980, 13, 44, 151
  Housing Act 1985, 151
  Housing Act 1996, 139
  and independent living, 143–4
  and mental health, 153–4,
     Australia, Denmark, New Zealand,
     Sweden, USA, 160
  special needs housing, 138, 139, 154
Hoyes, L., 86, 124
Hudson, B., 64, 94
Hughes, B., 112, 114, 119, 122
Hugman, R., 112, 127, 128, 190
Humphreys, B., 198, 203
Humphreys, S., 137
Hunter, D., 54, 57
Husband, C., 180

ideology, women and family, 164–6
independent living, 136–9, 143–4
  independent living movement, 139,
     142, 146
  Belgium, Denmark, European
     Commission, France, Italy,
     Netherlands, 143–4
  Canada, service brokerage, 144
  USA, 161
informal family care, 8, 9, 24, 38, 43,
     79–80, 164–8, 176, 177, 207

invalid care allowance, 171, 172
Irwin, S., 11
Itzen, C., 114

Jack, A., 48
Jackson, B., 5
James, A., 102
Jary, D. and J., 18
Jerrome, D., 113
Jessop, B., 11
Jewish Care, London, 186
Johnson, J., 114
Johnson, N., 43, 44, 59
Johnson, P., 111
Jones, C., 103
Jones, D., 117
Jones, K., 33, 35, 38, 39, 40, 41, 44, 47
Jones, S., 33

Keith, L., 133, 138
Kember, M., 18, 177
Kent, I., 156
Kerans, P., 19
Keynes, John Maynard, 35, 36
Kingdom, E., 202
Klein, R., 37, 54
Knowles, C., 71
Kohler, M., 124
KPMG Peat Marwick, 124

Labour, new govt., xiv, 7, 60, 68, 143,
     201, 205, 209, 210
Laing, R. D., 67
Land, H., 165
Langan, M., 86
Lart, R., 124
Lash, S., 12, 14
Laslett, P., 112
Lavalette, M., 25, 43
Law, I., 99, 181, 183, 184, 191
Lawson, R., 85
Leach, B., 141, 142
learning disabilities, people with,
     40–1, 136–7
  All-Wales Strategy, 137
  *Better Services for the Mentally
     Handicapped* (1971), 40
  eugenics and Nazi social policy, 33,
     136, 189

Lee, P., 28
Leff, J., 75
Le Grand, J., 15, 56, 60
Leonard, P., 25
Lewis, J., 61, 62, 63, 78, 79, 86, 88, 89, 90, 92, 94, 96, 100, 101, 167, 172, 173
liberalism, 27, 46
Lindow, V., 157, 159, 161
Lipietz, A., 11
Lipsedge, M., 71
Lister, R., 140, 195
Littlewood, R., 71
Loader, B., 76
Local Authority Act 1970, 41
Local Authority Social Services Act 1968, 38
Local Government Act 1929, 34
Local Government Reorganisation Act 1974, 39
Local Government and Housing Act 1990, 44
Lockwood, J., 152
Lodziak, C., 7
long-term care, funding of, 123–4
Lonsdale, S., 132, 141, 143
Lorenz, W., 104
Lowe, R., 37, 38, 41, 43
Lowry, S., 149
Lunacy Act 1845, 29
   Royal Commission, 1924, 33
Lund, B., 139, 151, 152, 163
Lunt, N., 94
Luthra, M., 182

Macdonald, K. M., 51
MacIntyre, A., 200
Maclean, M., 18
McCabe, D., 139
McEwen, E., 111, 121
McGarvey, N., 86
McGrath, M., 137
McLauglin, E., 127
McNally, S., 77
Major, John, 45, 57
Malin, N., 84
Malpass, P., 151
Maltby, T., 129

Mama, A., 182
managerialism, xiv, xv, 16–17, 23, 43, 44, 46, 51, 54–8, 74, 76, 85, 101, 102, 103, 158, 196, 205, 208
Manchester Jewish Social Services, 186
Mandlestam, M., 107
Manthorpe, J., 79, 80
Marshall, J., 200
Marshall, T. H., xiii, 193, 195, 196
Massey, D., 84
Means, R., 34, 45, 61, 62, 68, 70, 73, 83, 84, 86, 94, 104, 124, 144, 153, 163
Medicaid and Medicare, 73, 104, 190
mental disorder, nature of, 65
Mental Health Act 1959, 39
   Commission on Mental Illness & Mental Deficiency, 1959, 39
   Better Services for the Mentally Ill (1975), 39, 69
Mental Health Act 1983, 69, 149
mental health services, organisation of, 69
   and racism, 70–1
   Italy, 73
Mental Health (Patients in the Community) Act 1996, 156
Mental Illness Specific Grant, 70
Meredith, B., 50, 61, 70, 79, 87, 88, 89, 92, 94, 96, 99, 102
Meredith, B., 167, 172, 173
Merseyside Jewish Welfare Council, 187
Midwinter, A., 86
Midwinter, E., 30, 31, 32, 37, 38, 41, 42, 44
Mill, J. S., 27, 30
Millar, J., 171
Miller, S. 43
MIND (National Association for Mental Health), 69, 156, 157
Mirza, K., 182, 183
Mishra, R., 126
Modood, T., 182, 185, 191
Mohan, J., 53, 57, 60, 75
Moore, W., 155
Morris, J., 133, 138, 141, 147, 174

Morris, L., 11
Morrison, E., 133
Muijen, M., 154
Mulgan, G., 201
Munn-Giddings, C., 116
Murie, A., 44, 151, 160
Murphy, E., 29, 30, 33, 39, 65, 69, 70, 156, 158

Nash, C., 125
National Assistance Act 1948, 38, 116, 117
Navarro, N., 72
needs assessment, 62
Newman, J., 16, 85
New Right, 13, 15, 16
  and neo-liberalism, 28–9, 43, 44, 45, 46, 47, 52, 59, 74, 76, 84, 103, 104, 106, 107, 151, 204
NHS Act 1946, 37
NHS and Community Care Act 1990, 83–4, 119
NHS Review 1988, 52
Nicholls, V., 90
Nixon, J., 101
Nocon, A., 132, 134, 159
normalisation theory, 21, 40, 67, 136, 137
Norman, A., 115
Nozick, R., 200

Ogg, J., 116
O'Kell, S., 123
Okin, S. M., 165
Oliver, D., 193, 195, 196
Oliver, J., 135
Oliver, M., 21, 29, 115, 130, 131, 132, 133, 134, 141, 145, 146, 147, 195
Oppenheim, C., 121, 122, 123, 135, 136
O'Sullivan, N., 28
Owen, D., 113

Parker, G., 140
participation, 138, 197–207
Pascall, G., 18
Patel, N., 113, 115, 117, 181

Patients' Charters, 54
Paul, S., 106
Payne, M., 80, 84, 97, 98, 99, 103
Payne, S., 131, 135, 152
Peace, S., 112
Pensions Act 1929, 34
Pensions Act 1937, 34
Pensions Act 1995, 121
Petch, A., 153
Peters, M., 200
Pfeifer, D., 137
Pharoah, C., 117
Philpott, T., 107
physical impairment and built environment, 134–6, 170
Pickup, I., 170
Pickvance, C., 11
Pierson, C., 12, 46
Pilcher, J., 111
Pilgrim, D., 48, 68, 154, 158, 159
Plant, R., 4, 14, 193, 195
post-Fordism, 11–14, 45, 46, 76, 102, 205
power and empowerment, 197–9, 207
Pratt, A., 25, 43
Professional Social Work, 123
psychiatry profession, 66, 67, 68, 70, 71, 156, 159
  Italy, 73
Public Health Act 1848, 30
purchaser:provider split, 19, 20, 52, 53, 56, 63, 76–7, 86, 87–9, 100, 120, 196, 198, 203, 205, 209

quality assurance and social work, 102, 157
quasi-markets, 56, 60, 63, 64, 86, 101, 158, 196, 200, 201, 203, 205, 208, 209
quangos, 199
Qureshi, H., 113, 132, 134, 159

Raban, C., 28
Race, D., 131
racial discrimination and racism, 179–81
  Aliens Act 1905, 180
  Commission for Racial Equality, 180

racial discrimination and racism
(*continued*)
  and community care services, 181–3,
    207
  and mental health, 70–1, 181
  and welfare
    Germany, 190
    Sweden, 189
    USA, 190
  Race Relations Act 1976, 189
Rack, P., 71
Rai, D. K., 122, 123, 184
Ramcharan, P., 203
Rao, N., 87
Rawls, J., 200
Reading, P., 89, 90, 91
Redmond, E., 117
Rees, A., 37
Registered Homes Act 1984, 78, 118
Renshaw, J., 68, 69, 70, 137
residential care, 78, 174
  Residential Home Act 1980, 118
Resource Allocation Working Party
    (RAWP), 60
Reuler, J., 161
Rimmer, L., 170
Ritchie, P., 102
Roberts, H., 165
Rogers, A., 48, 154, 158, 159
Rogers, S., 152
Rose, J., 77
Roskill, C., 188
Rostron, J., 138
Rowe, A., 138
Runneymede Commission on Anti-
    Semitism, 188
Ryan, J., 21, 33, 41, 67, 136

Sahlin, I., 160
Sainsbury, D., 177
Salisbury, B., 144
Saltman, B., 54
Sampson, C., 18
Sandel, M., 200
Sandvin, J. T., 143
Sashidharan, S., 71
Sassoon, M., 159
Saunders, S., 170

schizophrenia, 149, 150, 154–6, 157
  and single homeless, 150
  Clunis, Christopher, 155
  National Schizophrenia Fellowship
    (NSF), 69, 157
Schmool, M., 178
Schwer, B., 107
Scrutton, S., 114, 116
Scull, D., 68
Seddon, J., 143
Seebohm Report, 38, 40, 41
Sen, K., 112
Sexty, C., 152
Shakespeare, T., 141
Shapiro, J., 64
Shonfield, A., 37
Siim, B., 127, 175
Sim, D., 191
Simic, P., 68
Skellington, R., 71, 183
Skidmore, D., 4, 6, 14, 75
Slater, P., 126
Smith, H., 133
Smith, R., 34, 45, 61, 62, 68, 70, 73,
    83, 84, 86, 94, 104, 144, 153,
    163
Snell, J., 105
social democracy, 193
social movements
  Australia, 125,
  National Pensioners' Convention,
    125
  Older Women's Project, 125
  USA, 125
social role valorisation, 67
  see also normalisation
Social Security Act 1986, 44
Social Services Inspectorate, 182
social workers, and care management,
    99–100
  occupational stress, 102
socialism, 32
Solomos, J., 180
South, N., 18
Spicker, P., 153
state collectivism, 30–1, 34–5, 36
Stevenson, J., 35
Strong, S., 157

Stuart, O., 115
Sturges, P. J., 100
Sullivan, M., 37, 43, 47, 54, 58, 59, 76
Swithibank, A., 105
Szasz, T., 67

Tawney, R. H., 28
Taylor, C., 200
Taylor, D., 194
Taylor, M., 89, 197
Taylor-Gooby, P., 59, 105, 107
Tester, S., 72, 73, 104, 106, 126, 127, 129, 175, 176, 190
Thain, J., 125
Thane, P., 34
Thatcherism, 42–6
Thomas, F., 21, 33, 41, 67, 136
Timmins, N., 37
Timms, P., 149, 150, 154
Tinker, A., 117, 118, 119, 129
Tomlinson, D., 161, 163
Tonnies, F., 5
Townsend, P., 19, 30, 39, 111
Twigg, J., 165, 168, 175
Tyne, A., 40, 145

Unemployed Assistance Board 1934, 33
Ungerson, C., 18, 165, 166, 168, 173, 177
United Kingdom Advocacy Network, 157
Urry, J., 12, 14
User empowerment, 157–9, 197–9
    African-Caribbean and Asian user groups, 159
    involvement and citizenship, 194–6, 206
    Psychiatric Survivors' Movement, 157, 159
    self-help movement, Canada, USA, 161

Valios, N., 92, 137
Vernon, S., 132, 133, 135, 141, 145, 147
voluntary sector, 9, 19, 22, 23, 31, 32, 36, 38, 47, 69, 89–90, 104, 107, 204, 209

and citizenship, 195, 201, 202
and minority ethnic groups, 185–9
    black organisations, 91–2, 185
    Chinese community, 188–9
    European Union, 105
    Jewish community, 186–8
for elderly persons, 119
women working in, 168–9, 176
Waerness, K., 127, 173
Wagner, Dame G., 139
Walby, S., 55
Walker, A., 45, 121, 129
Walker, R., 91, 183
Wall, A., 75
Walmsley, J., 141
Walzer, M., 200
Warde, A., 46
Watson, S., 152
Watters, C., 71
Weaver, M., 151
Weber, M., 4, 18
Weir, M., 190
Welch, C., 141
welfare state and ideology, 36–42
Wetherly, P., 7
White, C., 139
Whiteley, P., 92, 156
Whittaker, T., 116
Widows', Orphans' and Old Age Contributory Pensions Act 1925, 34
Wilding, P., 34, 35, 43
Williams, B., 186
Williams, F., 133, 169, 180
Williams, R., 4
Wilmott, P., 4, 5
Wilson, E., 35, 47, 170
Wilson, V., 143, 144, 145, 146
Wing, H., 102
Wistow, G., 61, 63, 86, 87, 90, 96
Wolfensburger, W., 67, 136, 137
women and caring, 16, 166–9, 176
    Eastern Europe, France, Germany, Netherlands, Scandinavia, 176
women and environment, 169–70
women and financial hardship, 170–2
    pensions, occupational, 171, 173
    pensions, widow's, 171, 173

women and financial hardship
    (*continued*)
  poverty and social security, 171
women and health, 172–3
'Working For Patients', White Paper
    (1989), 52–4, 74, 116

Wright, A., 28
Wright, K., 147

Young, M., 5
Yuval-Davis, N., 4

Zarb, G., 115